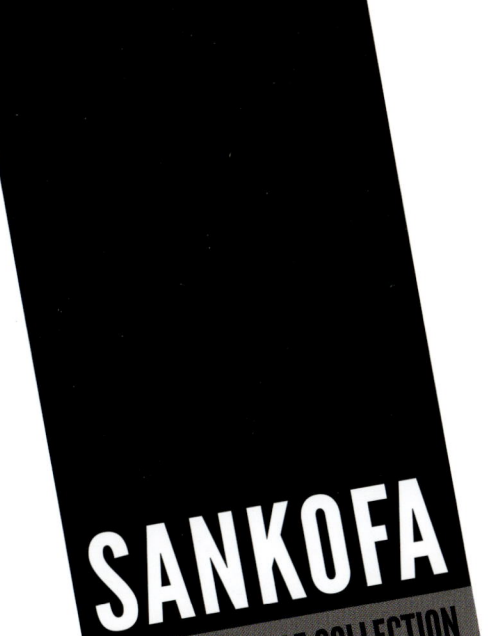

# SANKOFA
## BLACK HERITAGE COLLECTION

# SPORTING LIFE

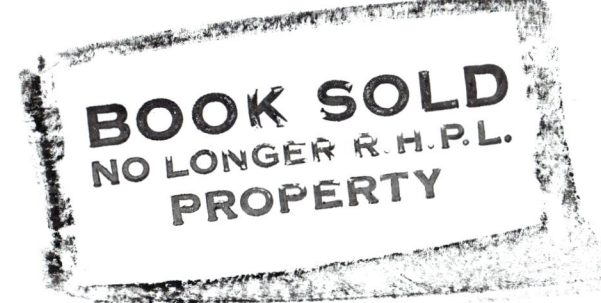
## PHILIP GIBSON

### SERIES EDITOR • TOM HENDERSON

**Ru'bicon**
www.rubiconpublishing.com

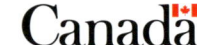

Funded by the
Government
of Canada | Canada

Associate Publisher: Amy Land
Project Editor: Jessica Rose
Editorial Assistant: Kim Therriault
Creative Director: Jennifer Drew
Lead Designer: Sherwin Flores
Graphic Designers: Roy Casim, Jennifer Harvey, Robin Lindner, Megan Little

Every reasonable effort has been made to trace the owners of copyrighted
material and to make due acknowledgement. Any errors or omissions
drawn to our attention will be gladly rectified in future editions.

21  22  23  24  25      8  7  6  5  4

ISBN: 978-1-77058-826-4

*Printed in China*

# CONTENTS

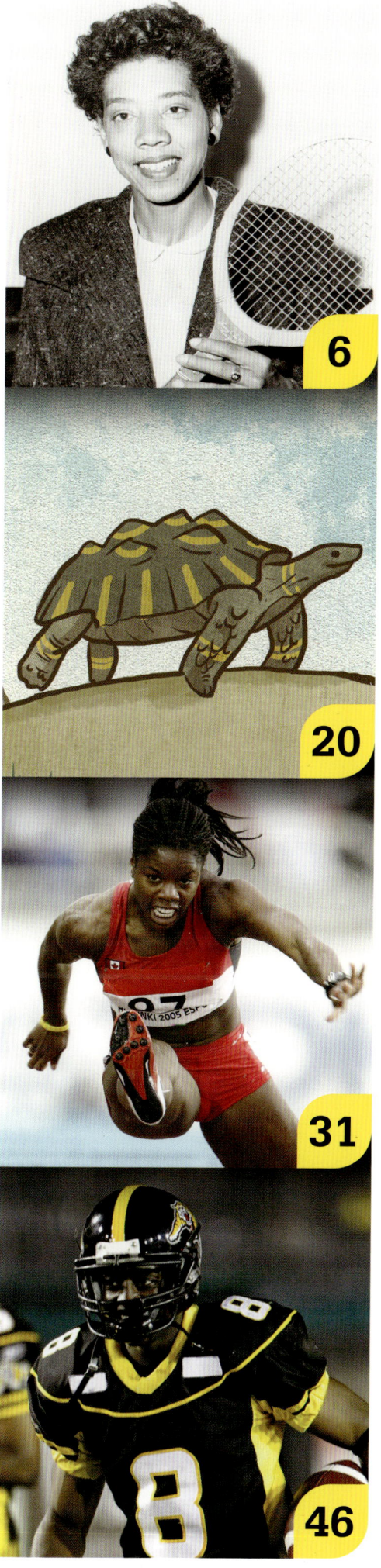

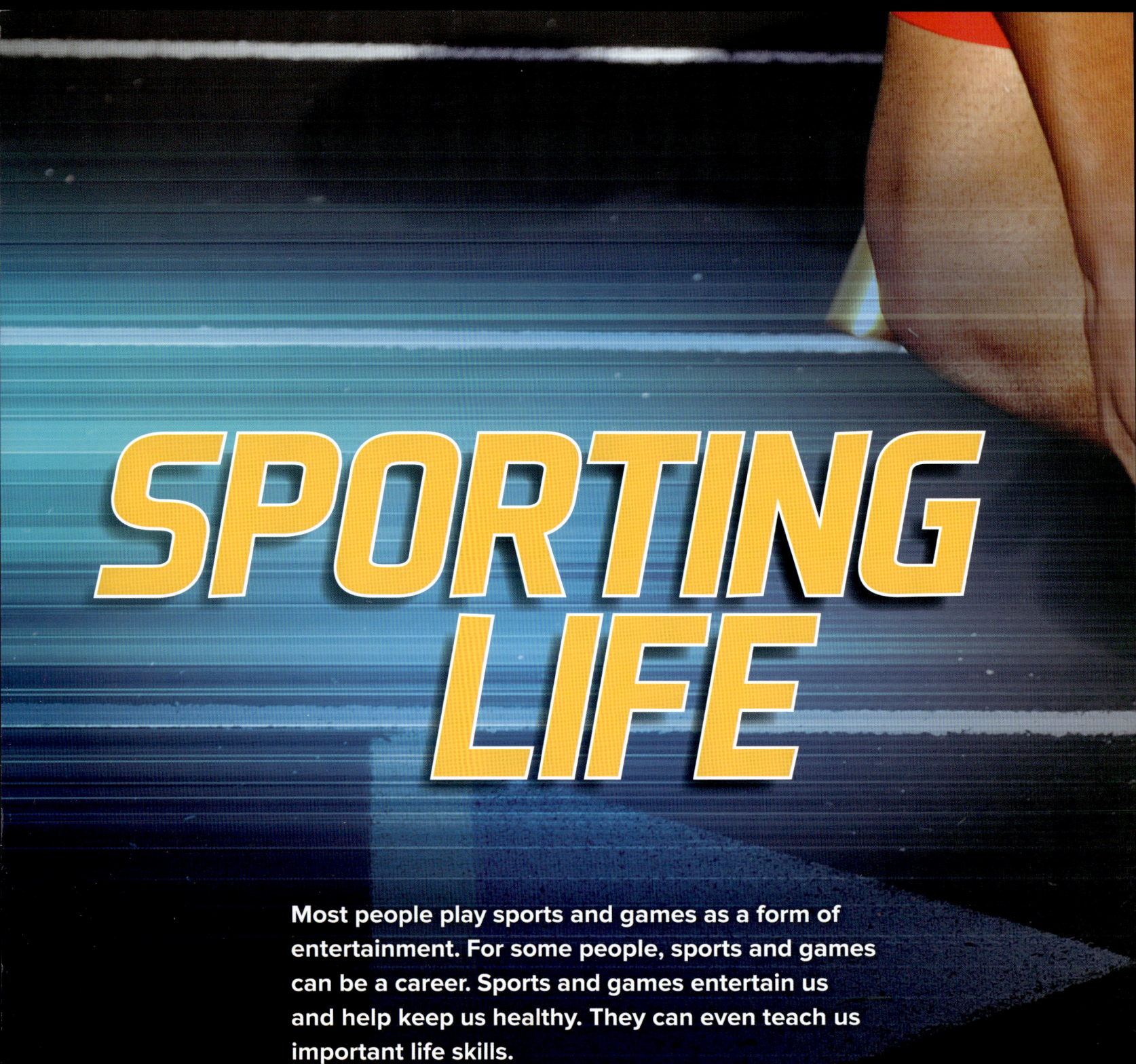

# SPORTING LIFE

Most people play sports and games as a form of entertainment. For some people, sports and games can be a career. Sports and games entertain us and help keep us healthy. They can even teach us important life skills.

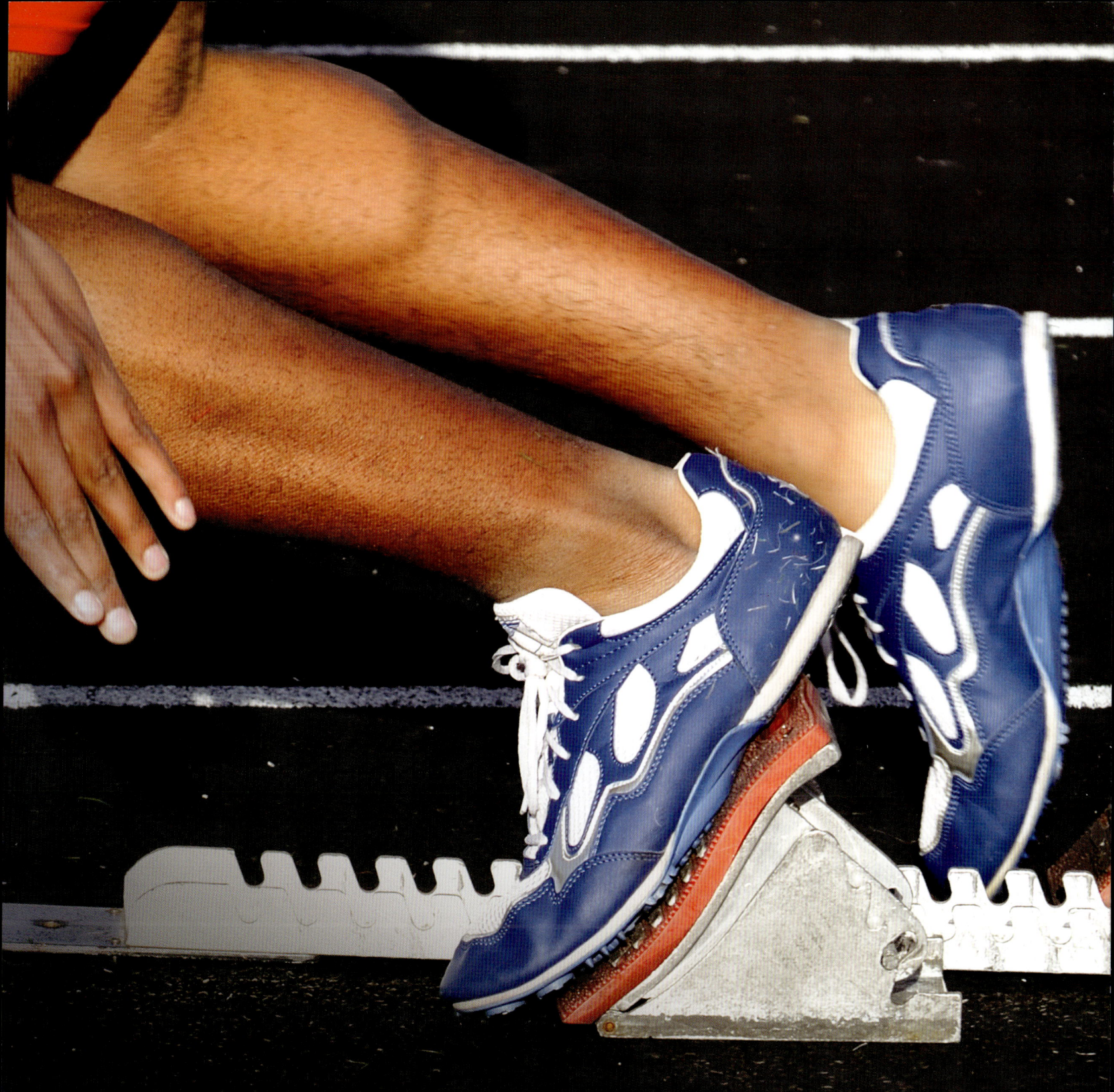

# How do sports and games improve our lives?

# KEY EVENTS IN
# SPORTING

### THINK ABOUT IT

How do you think sports have changed in the last 100 years? What changes might happen in the future?

**AMAZING ATHLETES WITH** incredible abilities have been breaking down the "colour barrier" in sports for over 100 years. Read about just a few of these athletes in this timeline.

Nova Scotia's George Dixon becomes the first Black man to win a world boxing title.

**1890**

Lucy Diggs Slowe becomes the first African American woman to win a national title in any sport. She wins the women's title at the American Tennis Association tournament.

**1917**

The Savoy Big Five basketball team is formed. It is a way for Black athletes to earn money while playing basketball. At the time, only White players can play professional basketball. In a few years, the team is renamed the Harlem Globetrotters.

**1926**

**1894**

The Coloured Hockey League of the Maritimes is created. The league's headquarters are in Halifax, Nova Scotia.

**1921**

The all-Black Halifax Coloured Diamonds baseball team wins the provincial coloured championships.

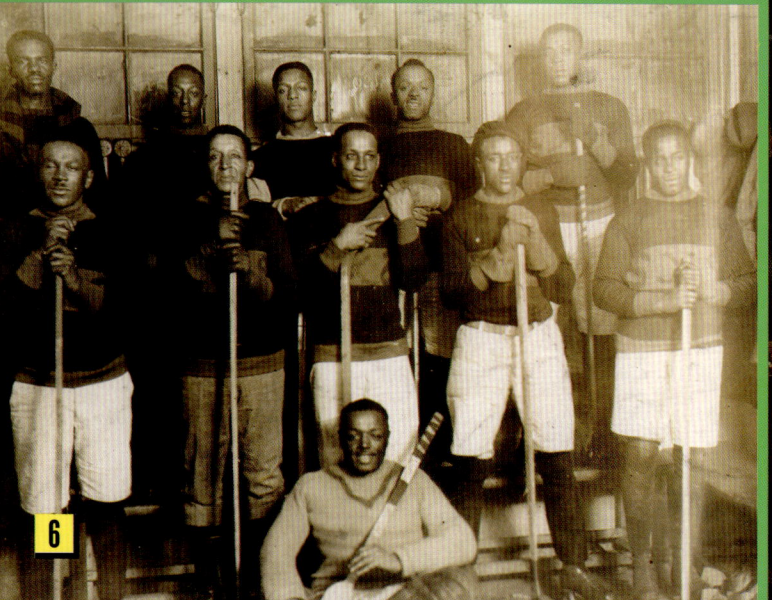

# HISTORY

Jackie Robinson starts his career playing for the Montreal Royals. He later goes on to change the face of baseball when he becomes the first Black athlete to play baseball in the major leagues.

## 1946

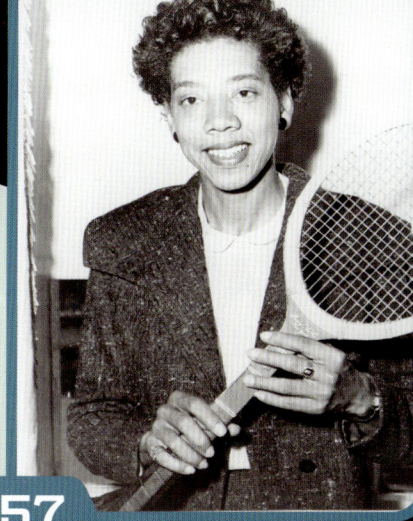

Althea Gibson wins the French Open, Wimbledon, and the US Open.

## 1956-57

## 1936

Jesse Owens becomes the first American track and field athlete to win four gold medals in one Olympiad at the Summer Olympics in Berlin.

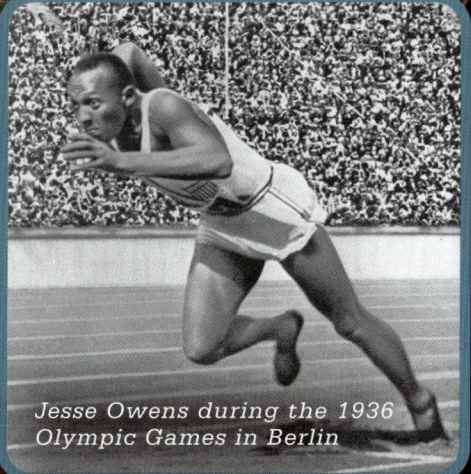

*Jesse Owens during the 1936 Olympic Games in Berlin*

## 1951

The University of San Francisco football team declines an invitation to play in the Orange Bowl in support of their two African American teammates who were not allowed to play.

## 1958

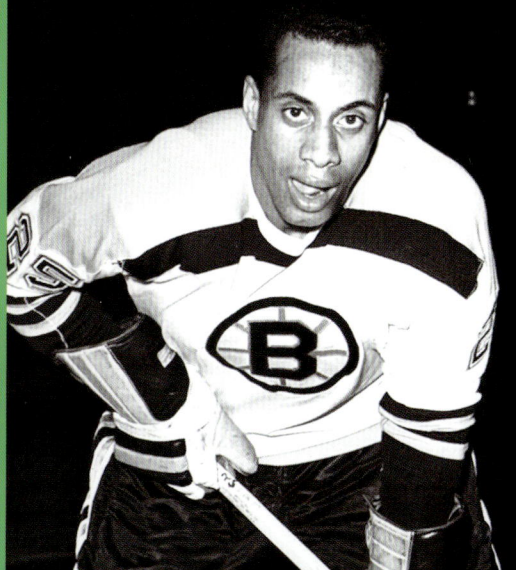

Willie O'Ree, who was born in Fredericton, New Brunswick, becomes the first Black man to play in the National Hockey League (NHL).

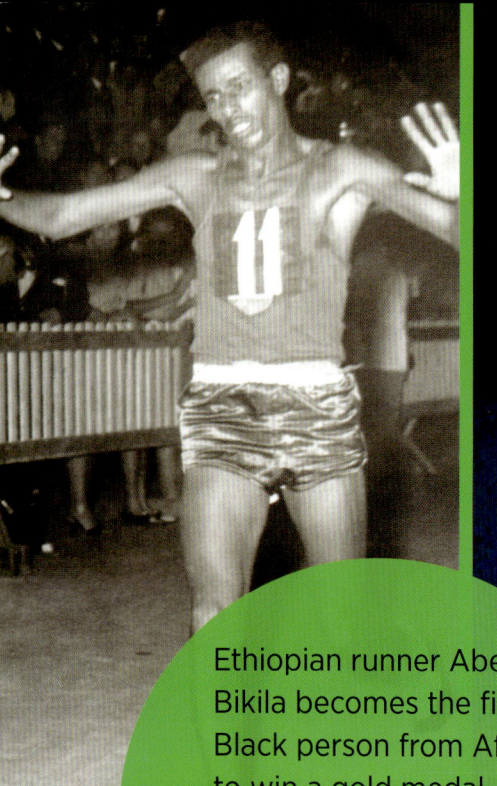

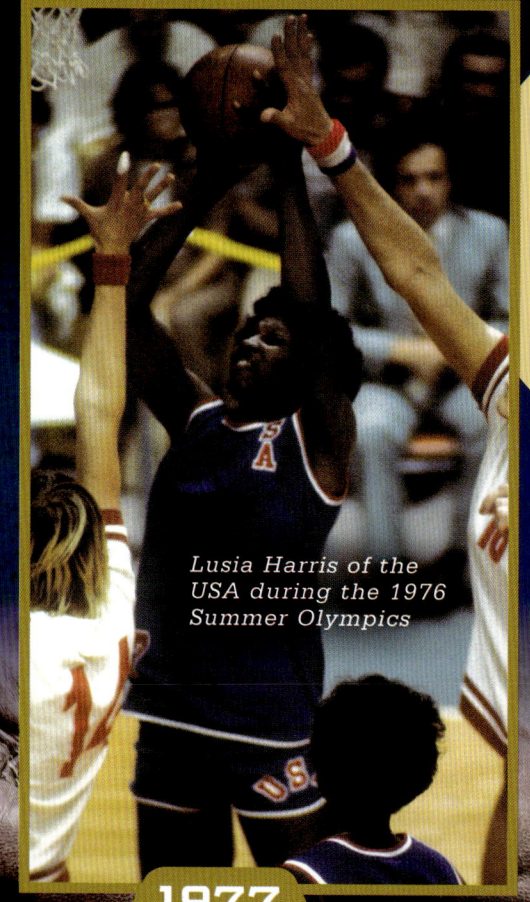

Lusia Harris, an African American basketball player, becomes the first woman ever to be drafted into the all-male National Basketball Association (NBA). She declines.

*Lusia Harris of the USA during the 1976 Summer Olympics*

Ethiopian runner Abebe Bikila becomes the first Black person from Africa to win a gold medal. This happens at the Olympic Games in Rome. He runs the entire race barefoot.

Tiger Woods becomes the first African American golfer to win the Masters Golf Tournament.

**1960**

**1977**

**1997**

**1961**

**1978**

Ernie Davis, a running back from Syracuse, New York, becomes the first African American to win the Heisman Trophy. This trophy is awarded to the most outstanding player in college football.

Muhammad Ali becomes the first boxer to win three heavyweight titles.

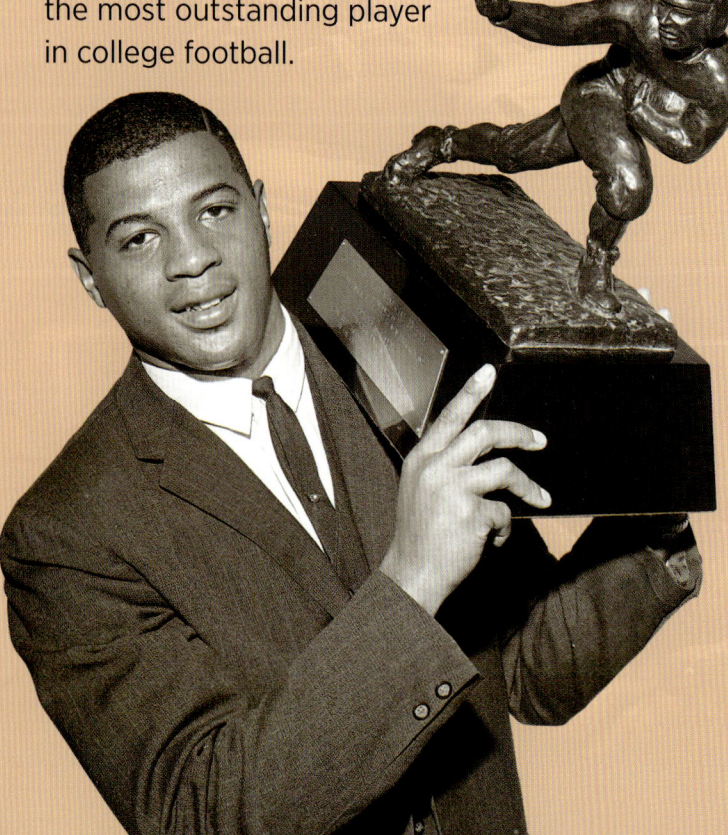

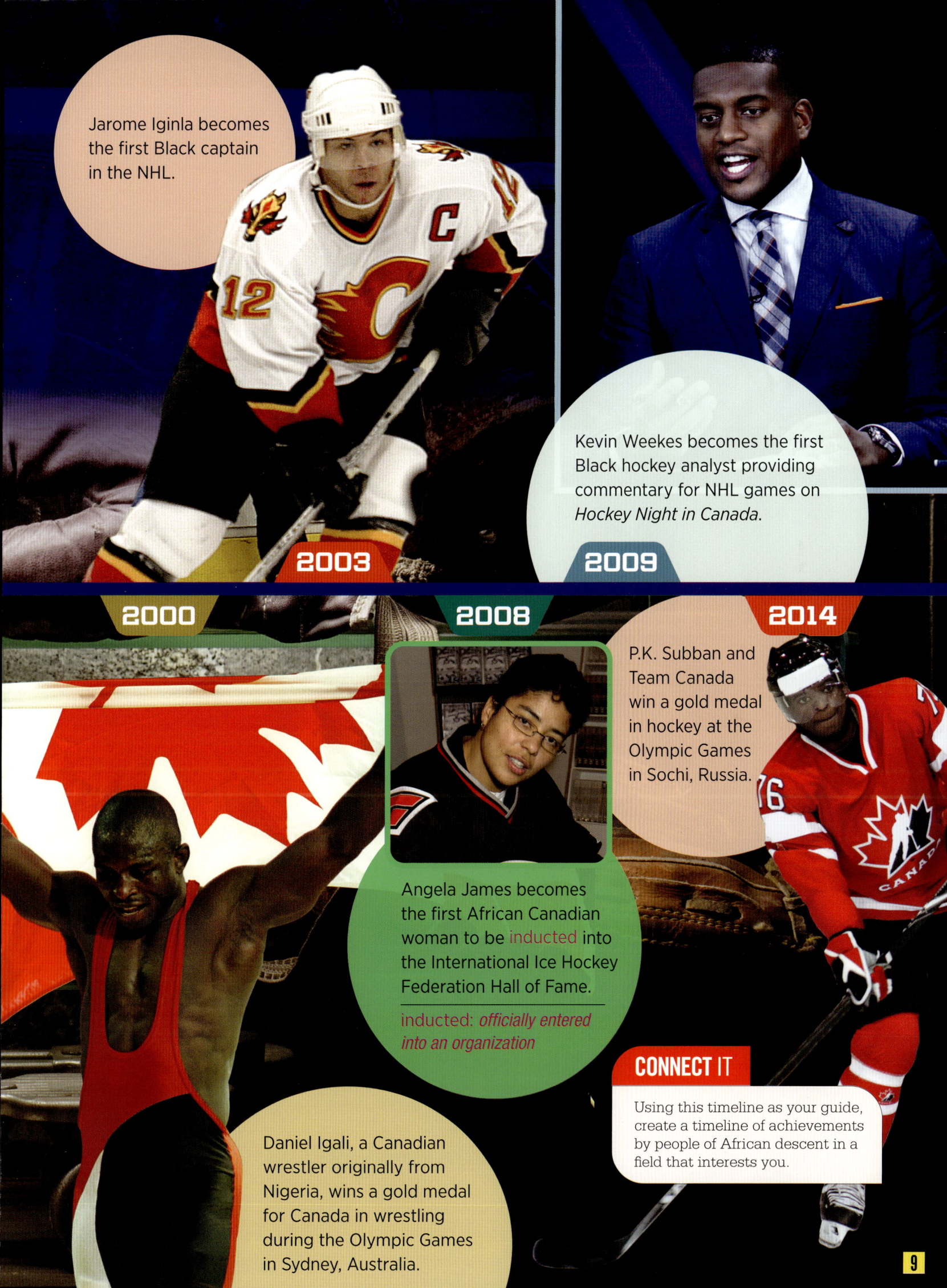

Jarome Iginla becomes the first Black captain in the NHL.

**2003**

Kevin Weekes becomes the first Black hockey analyst providing commentary for NHL games on *Hockey Night in Canada.*

**2009**

**2000**

**2008**

**2014**

P.K. Subban and Team Canada win a gold medal in hockey at the Olympic Games in Sochi, Russia.

Angela James becomes the first African Canadian woman to be inducted into the International Ice Hockey Federation Hall of Fame.

inducted: *officially entered into an organization*

Daniel Igali, a Canadian wrestler originally from Nigeria, wins a gold medal for Canada in wrestling during the Olympic Games in Sydney, Australia.

**CONNECT IT**

Using this timeline as your guide, create a timeline of achievements by people of African descent in a field that interests you.

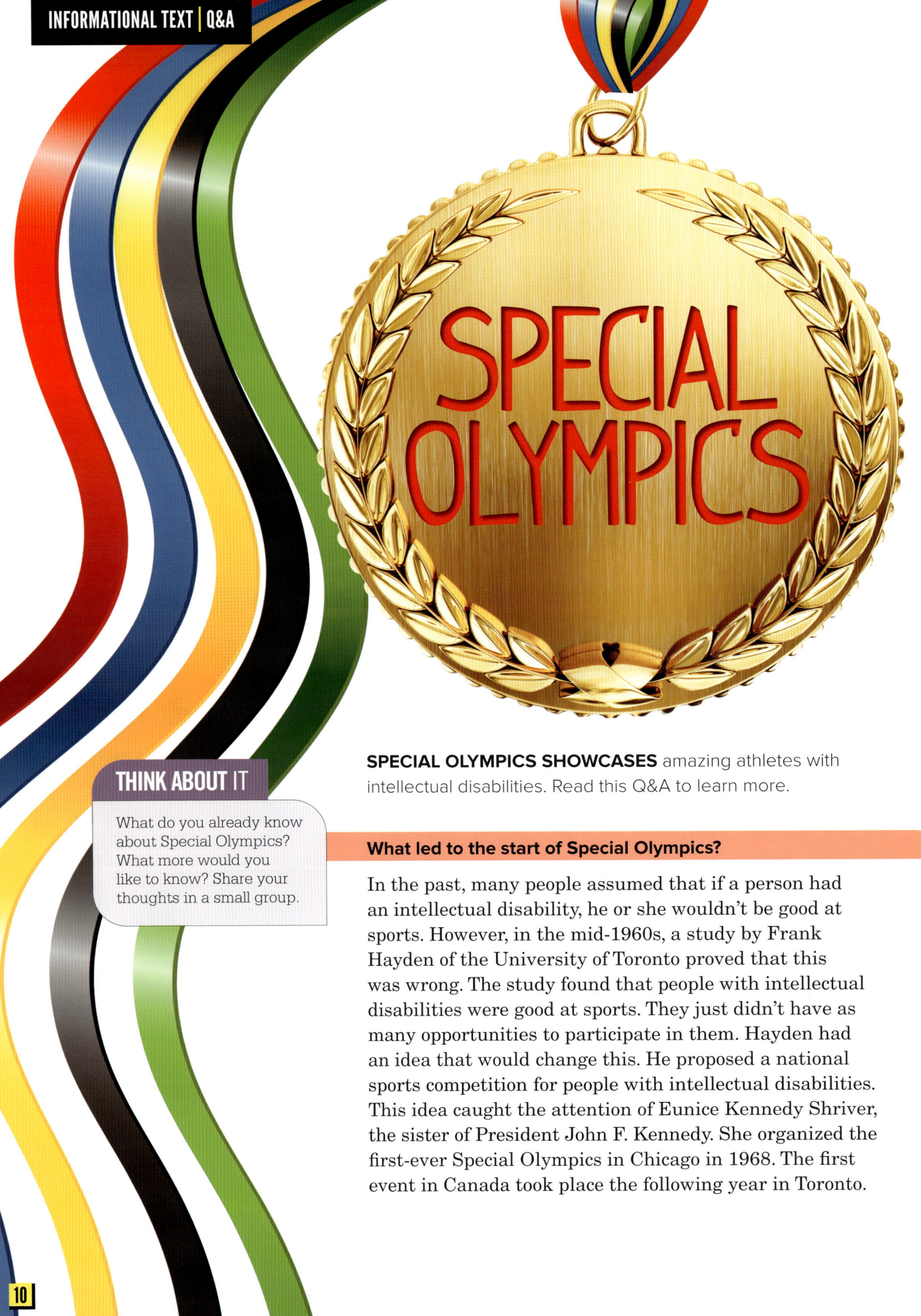

# SPECIAL OLYMPICS

**SPECIAL OLYMPICS SHOWCASES** amazing athletes with intellectual disabilities. Read this Q&A to learn more.

**THINK ABOUT IT**

What do you already know about Special Olympics? What more would you like to know? Share your thoughts in a small group.

## What led to the start of Special Olympics?

In the past, many people assumed that if a person had an intellectual disability, he or she wouldn't be good at sports. However, in the mid-1960s, a study by Frank Hayden of the University of Toronto proved that this was wrong. The study found that people with intellectual disabilities were good at sports. They just didn't have as many opportunities to participate in them. Hayden had an idea that would change this. He proposed a national sports competition for people with intellectual disabilities. This idea caught the attention of Eunice Kennedy Shriver, the sister of President John F. Kennedy. She organized the first-ever Special Olympics in Chicago in 1968. The first event in Canada took place the following year in Toronto.

## What is the difference between Special Olympics and Paralympics?

Special Olympics is for athletes with intellectual disabilities. Paralympics are for athletes with physical disabilities. Paralympics have an intellectual disability category. This means that Special Olympics athletes can also compete in the Paralympic Games, which take place every four years right after the Olympic Games.

## What are the Special Olympics World Games?

Every two years, Special Olympics hosts the Special Olympics World Games. The Games alternate between summer and winter events, and they're not only a sporting event but also a cultural and educational one. The Games have taken place in countries all over the world, including Ireland, Japan, Korea, Greece, and China. The Special Olympics Canada Games take place every two years. In 2014, they were held in Vancouver, British Columbia.

## What are some benefits of Special Olympics?

There are many benefits for athletes competing in Special Olympics. They include:

- greater self-confidence
- improved social skills
- better co-operation and leadership skills
- a sense of accomplishment

Special Olympics is committed to educating the public. It tries to change some of the negative ideas that exist about people with intellectual disabilities. Too often, the focus is on what people cannot do, rather than on what they can. Special Olympics helps to change that. It focuses on similarities between people, not differences.

*Torchbearers carry the torch for the Special Olympics Winter Games.*

**Who are some Special Olympics athletes?**

Read these fact cards about three Canadian Special Olympics athletes.

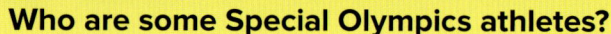

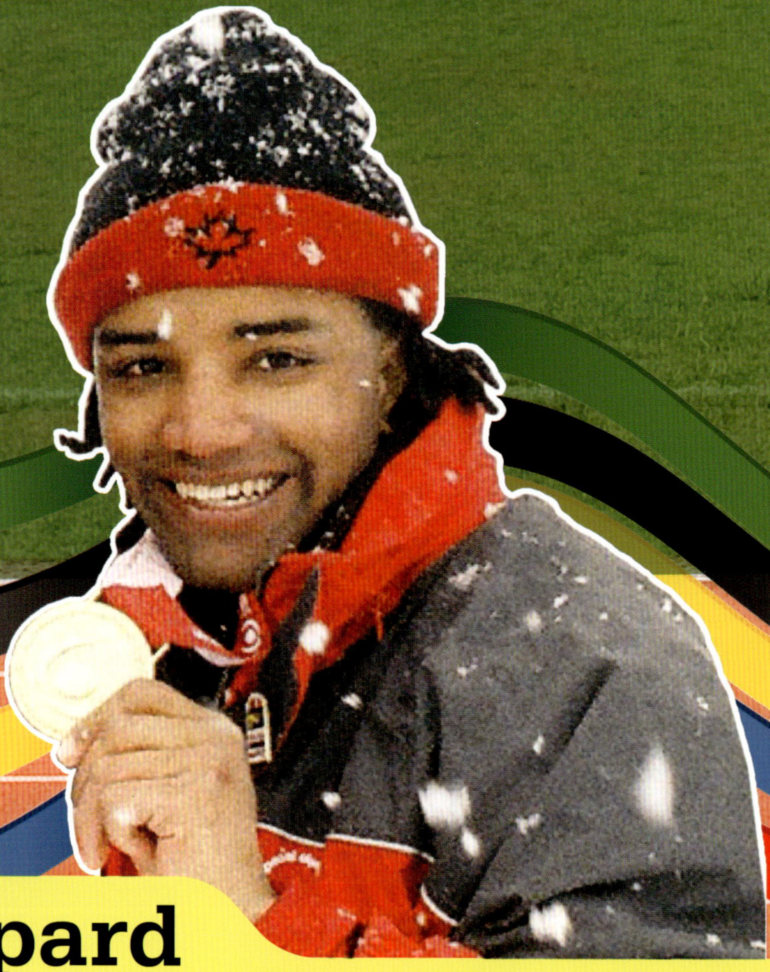

# Ian Sheppard

**Hometown:** Born in Manitoba, Sheppard now lives in Ontario.

**Sports:** Sheppard has competed in snowshoeing, cross country skiing, rugby, and track and field events.

**Medals:** Sheppard won three gold medals at the Special Olympics World Games in Nagano, Japan, and one gold medal in China.

**Quotation:** "Don't let anyone tell you you can't do it. In your heart, you know you can!"

**Interesting Facts:**

- One thing that Sheppard likes about Special Olympics is that all the athletes "get along really well. Everyone cheers and helps each other out."
- Sheppard enjoys running both the 200 m and 800 m races, but says it is nice to be able to "pace out your breath a bit more" in the 800 m.

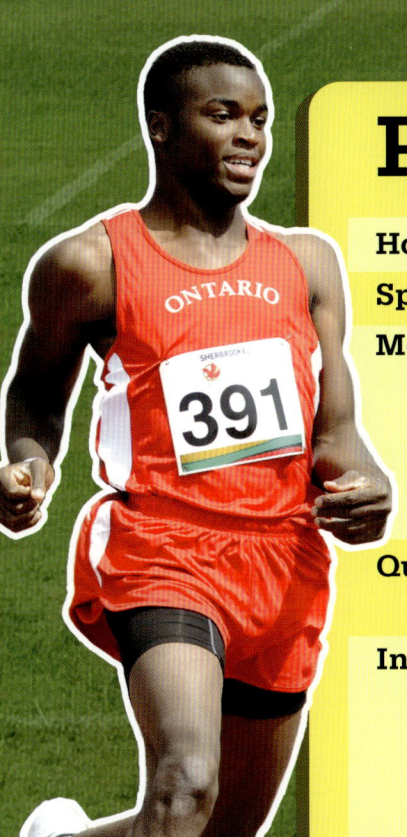

# Peter Snider

| | |
|---|---|
| **Hometown:** | Waterloo, Ontario |
| **Sports:** | Snider has competed in snowshoeing and track and field events. |
| **Medals:** | Snider won five gold medals at the 2013 Special Olympics Ontario Provincial Summer Games in track and field. He went on to win two gold medals (100 m and 200 m) at the Canada Summer Games. He won another gold at the 2013 Ontario Federation of School Athletic Associations (OFSAA). |
| **Quotation:** | "Training was hard, but I thought to myself, 'If I want to be on top, I need to do this.'" |

**Interesting Facts:**

- Snider's favourite memory is "when I crossed the finish line [at the Canada Games held in Sherbrooke, Quebec] and breathed a huge sigh of relief!"
- Snider loves the Toronto Raptors and playing Xbox. He loves fishing (practising catch and release), and he likes Usain Bolt.

# Monique Shah

| | |
|---|---|
| **Hometown:** | Edmonton, Alberta |
| **Sports:** | Some of the events Monique Shah has competed in include bowling, track and field, soccer, volleyball, and softball. |
| **Medals:** | She has won two gold medals in track and field at the 2011 Special Olympics World Summer Games in Athens, Greece. |
| **Quotation:** | "Don't give up. Try your best!" |

**Interesting Facts:**

- Shah once volunteered to play goalie for her soccer team at the 2003 Special Olympics World Summer Games in Ireland. Although she had never played that position before, she bravely said, "I'll give it a try!"
- Special Olympics has been an important part of Shah's life for almost 20 years. She used to have poor coordination and often bumped into doorways at school. That was before she was introduced to competitive sports.
- Shah's mother, June, explains that her daughter has "found a place where she's been accepted, formed lasting friendships, and met celebrities."

## CONNECT IT

Working in small groups, discuss the characteristics that these athletes have in common that helped them become successful.

# DIVERSITY
# IN THE NHL IS ON THE RISE

**JOHN VOGL**
*THE BUFFALO NEWS*
*26 JUNE 2013*

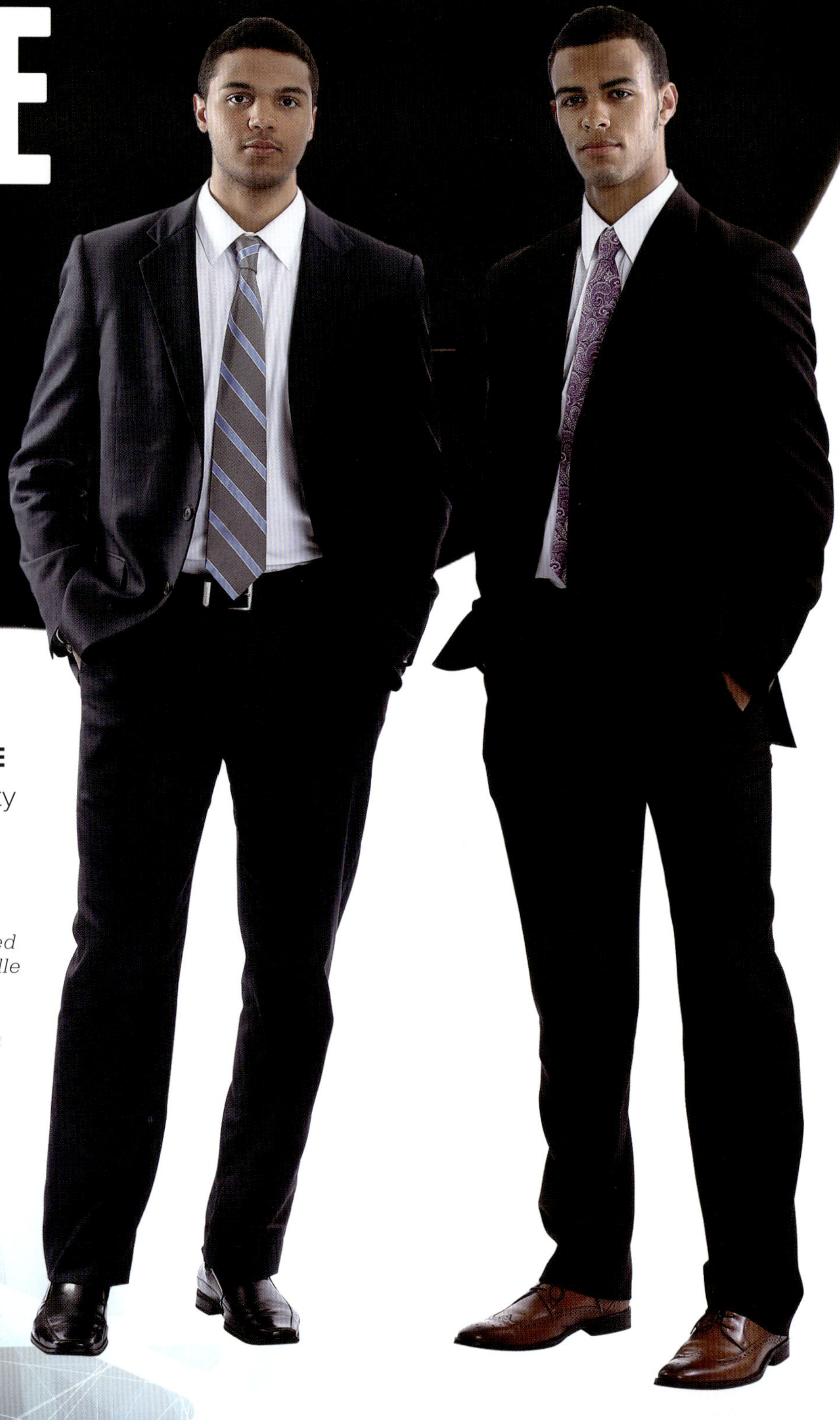

## THINK ABOUT IT

Why is diversity in sports important? Why do you think diversity is on the rise in the NHL?

**READ THIS NEWSPAPER ARTICLE**
to learn about how and why diversity is increasing in the NHL.

*Seth Jones (left) was selected fourth overall by the Nashville Predators in the 2013 NHL Entry Draft. Darnell Nurse (right) was selected seventh by the Edmonton Oilers.*

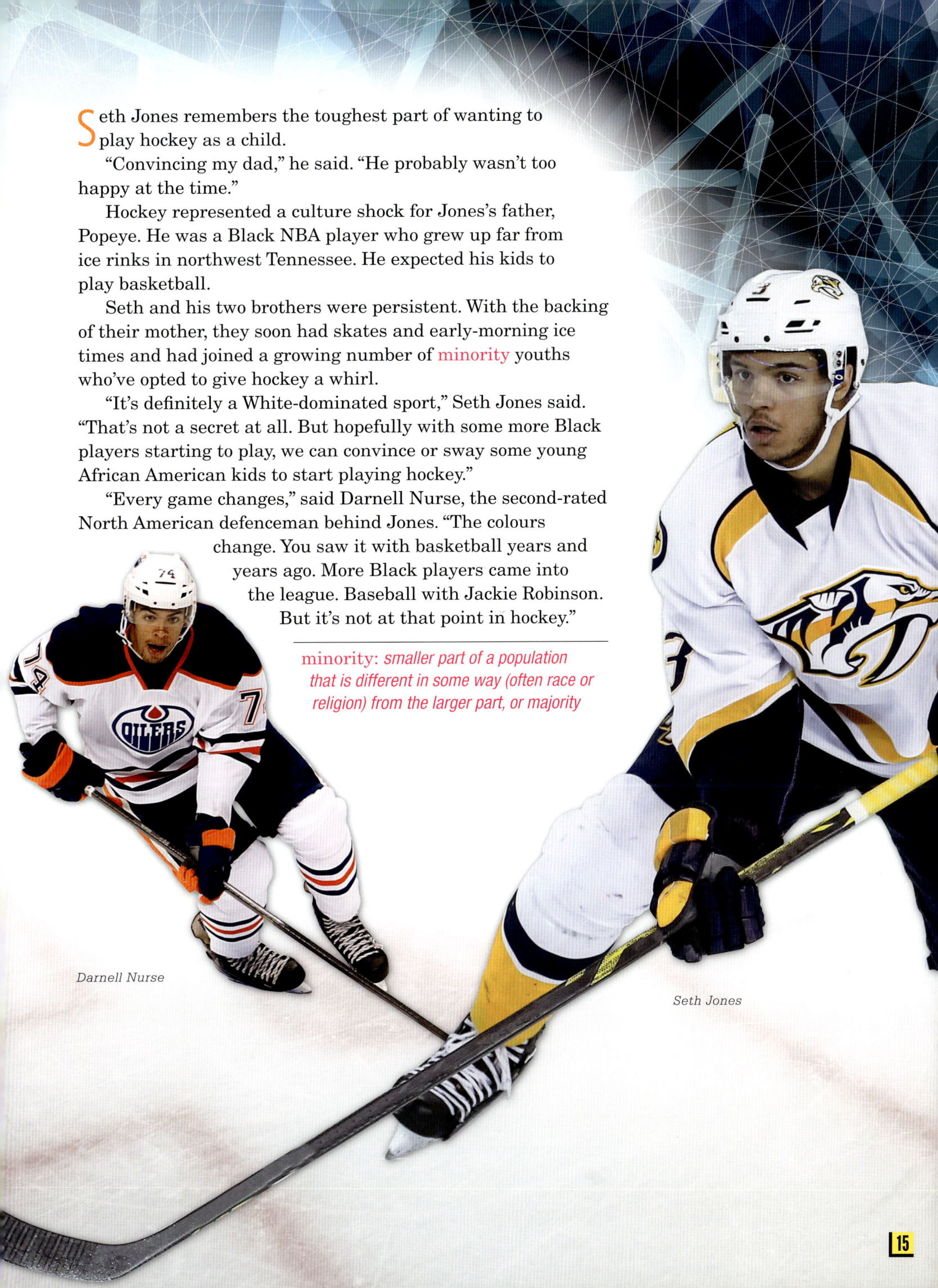

Seth Jones remembers the toughest part of wanting to play hockey as a child.

"Convincing my dad," he said. "He probably wasn't too happy at the time."

Hockey represented a culture shock for Jones's father, Popeye. He was a Black NBA player who grew up far from ice rinks in northwest Tennessee. He expected his kids to play basketball.

Seth and his two brothers were persistent. With the backing of their mother, they soon had skates and early-morning ice times and had joined a growing number of minority youths who've opted to give hockey a whirl.

"It's definitely a White-dominated sport," Seth Jones said. "That's not a secret at all. But hopefully with some more Black players starting to play, we can convince or sway some young African American kids to start playing hockey."

"Every game changes," said Darnell Nurse, the second-rated North American defenceman behind Jones. "The colours change. You saw it with basketball years and years ago. More Black players came into the league. Baseball with Jackie Robinson. But it's not at that point in hockey."

minority: *smaller part of a population that is different in some way (often race or religion) from the larger part, or majority*

Darnell Nurse

Seth Jones

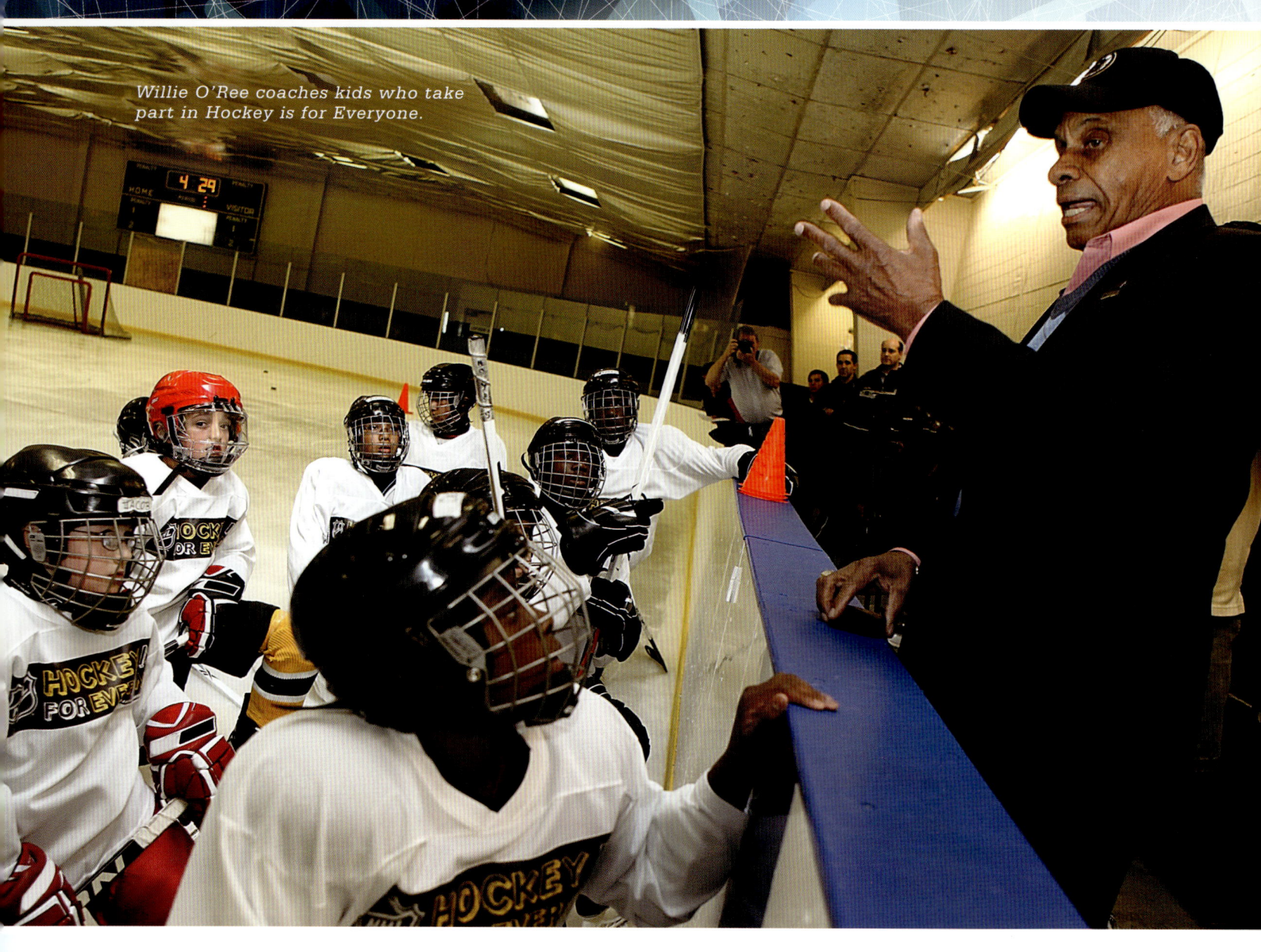

Willie O'Ree coaches kids who take part in Hockey is for Everyone.

The rise in minority participation has special meaning for Willie O'Ree. He became the NHL's first Black player in 1958, and is the ambassador for the league's Hockey is for Everyone initiative. …

"I can see more kids — not only kids of colour and Black kids, but more kids in general — getting into hockey and wanting to play this sport," O'Ree said by phone. …

Why do you think hockey is becoming more popular?

The NHL sponsors programs in 38 North American cities to help children of all backgrounds learn to play hockey. More than 45 000 boys and girls have been exposed to the sport through Hockey is for Everyone. …

Seth Jones says attending games was the toughest part for his father. A 6-foot-8 [203 cm] professional athlete would stand out anywhere, but that was particularly true in ice rinks.

"People would obviously give him weird looks and those sorts of things," said Jones, who eventually got his dad on the ice, but just once. "He did not let go of the boards. Literally, did not, grabbing the boards, pulling himself around the rink."

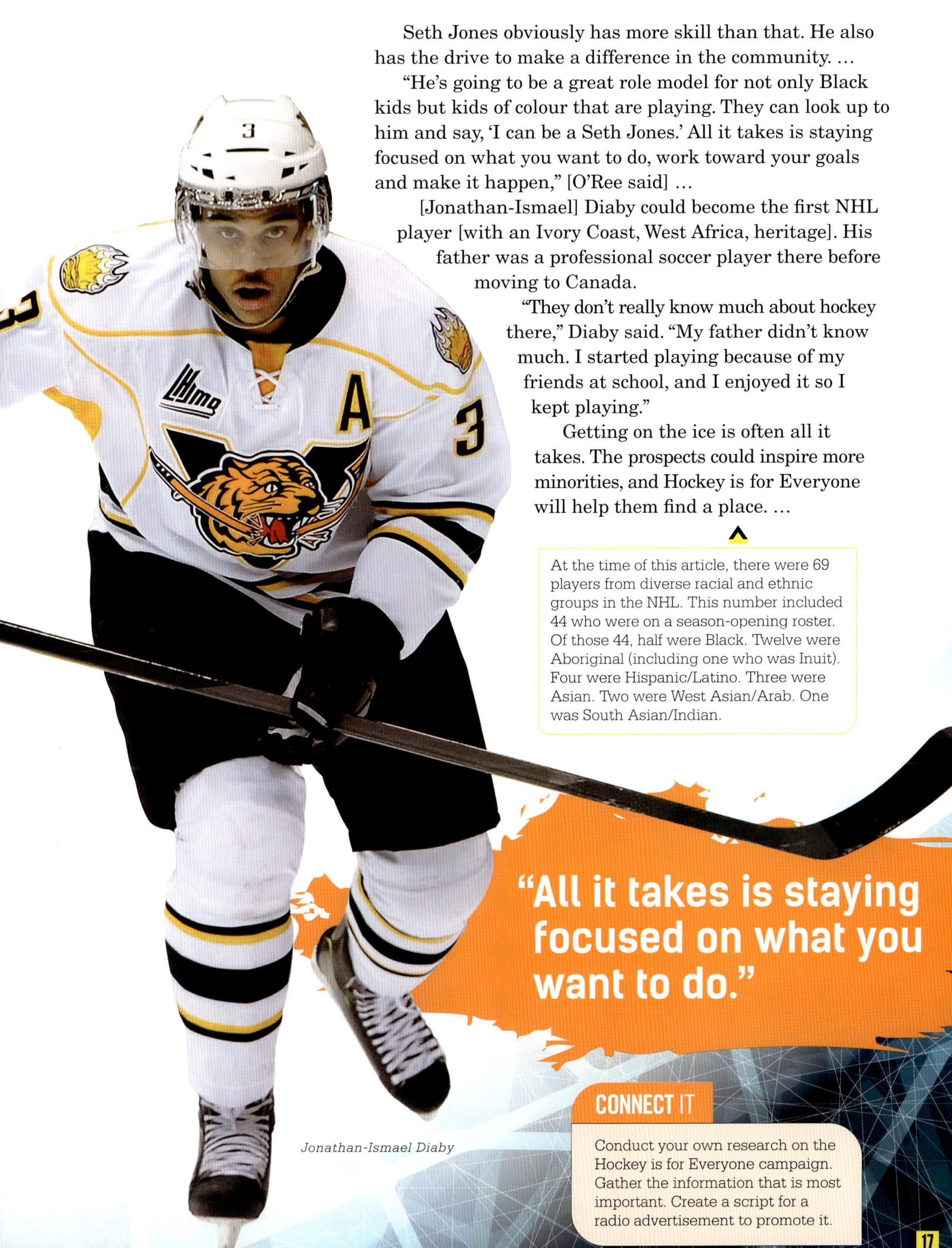

Seth Jones obviously has more skill than that. He also has the drive to make a difference in the community. …

"He's going to be a great role model for not only Black kids but kids of colour that are playing. They can look up to him and say, 'I can be a Seth Jones.' All it takes is staying focused on what you want to do, work toward your goals and make it happen," [O'Ree said] …

[Jonathan-Ismael] Diaby could become the first NHL player [with an Ivory Coast, West Africa, heritage]. His father was a professional soccer player there before moving to Canada.

"They don't really know much about hockey there," Diaby said. "My father didn't know much. I started playing because of my friends at school, and I enjoyed it so I kept playing."

Getting on the ice is often all it takes. The prospects could inspire more minorities, and Hockey is for Everyone will help them find a place. …

At the time of this article, there were 69 players from diverse racial and ethnic groups in the NHL. This number included 44 who were on a season-opening roster. Of those 44, half were Black. Twelve were Aboriginal (including one who was Inuit). Four were Hispanic/Latino. Three were Asian. Two were West Asian/Arab. One was South Asian/Indian.

Jonathan-Ismael Diaby

"All it takes is staying focused on what you want to do."

**CONNECT IT**

Conduct your own research on the Hockey is for Everyone campaign. Gather the information that is most important. Create a script for a radio advertisement to promote it.

# Tuesday

◖ **BY DIONNE BRAND**

### THINK ABOUT IT

If you had to spend a day with no computer and no television, how would you spend it? Would you like to have a day like this? Share your ideas in a small group.

Tuesday
light blue haze,
fat lady bug days,
in a sunlit maze.
Bruised knee spills
on San Fernando hill,
searching every street,
liking people that you meet,
step on a crack if you dare,
cross your fingers, wish in the air,
Sister says you shouldn't stray,
down that darkened alley way,
says don't stare, hurry home,
night may catch us all alone

◀ San Fernando is a city in Trinidad and Tobago.

haze: *dust or moisture in the air that makes it hard to see*
stray: *wander away*

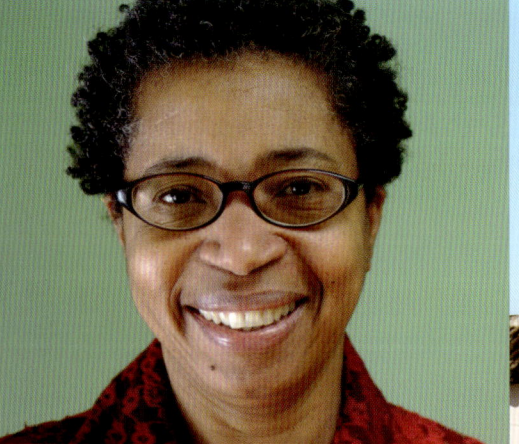

### ABOUT THE POET

Dionne Brand was born in Trinidad and Tobago in 1953. She moved to Toronto when she was 17. As a child, Brand loved spending time with a good book in her hiding space under her bed. Today, she is one of Canada's best-known poets. In 2009, she was named Toronto's Poet Laureate. She won the Griffin Poetry Prize in 2011.

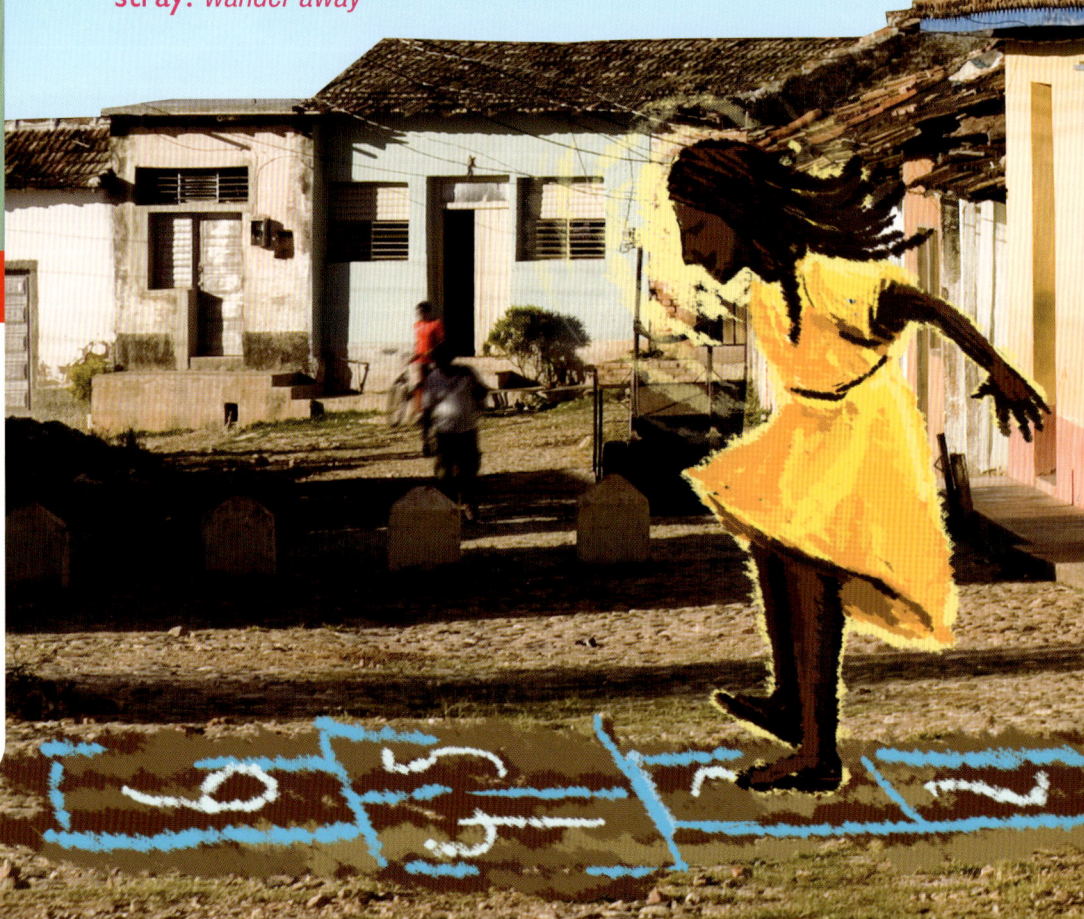

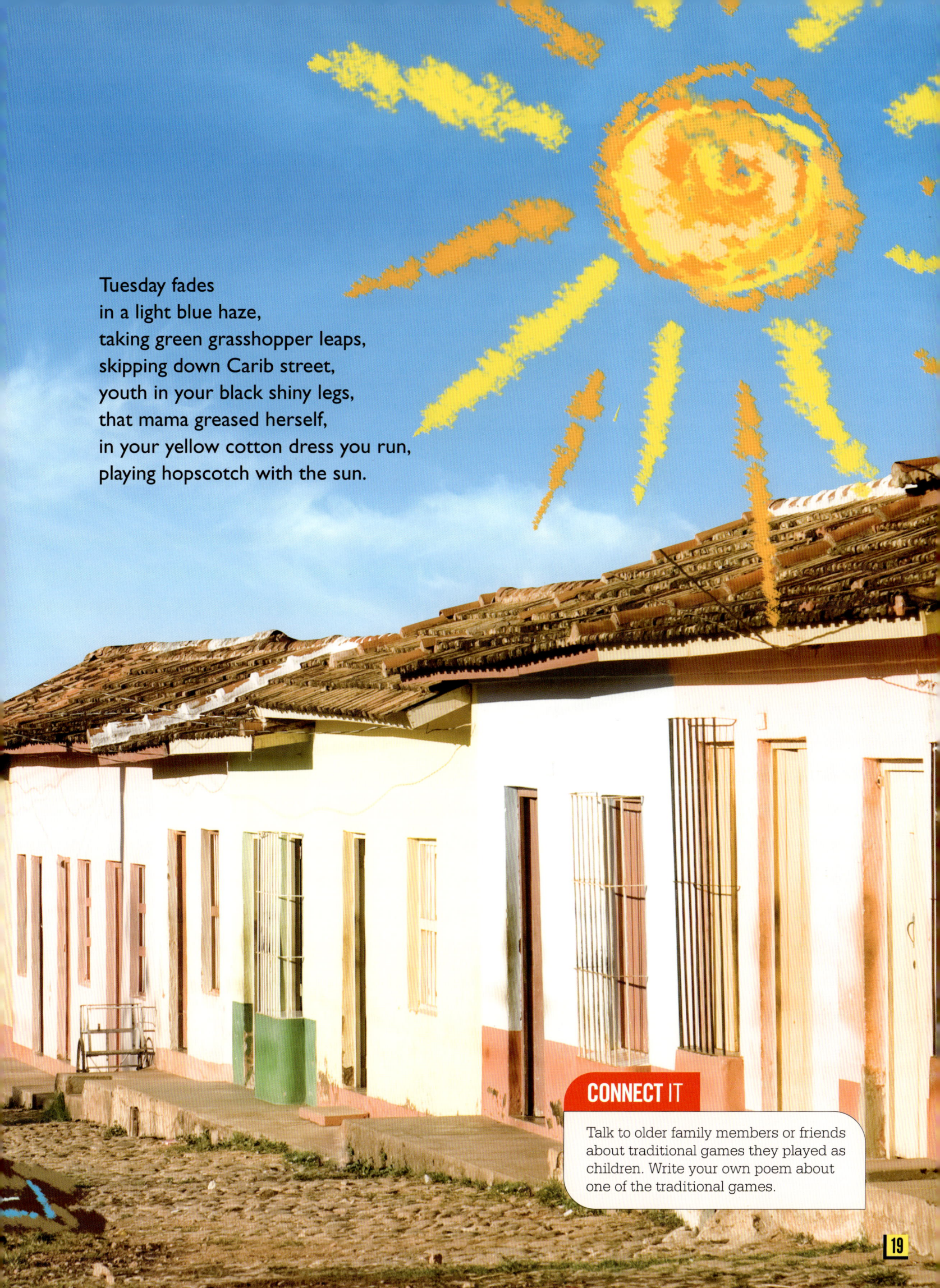

Tuesday fades
in a light blue haze,
taking green grasshopper leaps,
skipping down Carib street,
youth in your black shiny legs,
that mama greased herself,
in your yellow cotton dress you run,
playing hopscotch with the sun.

**CONNECT IT**

Talk to older family members or friends about traditional games they played as children. Write your own poem about one of the traditional games.

# THE TORTOISE AND THE RACE

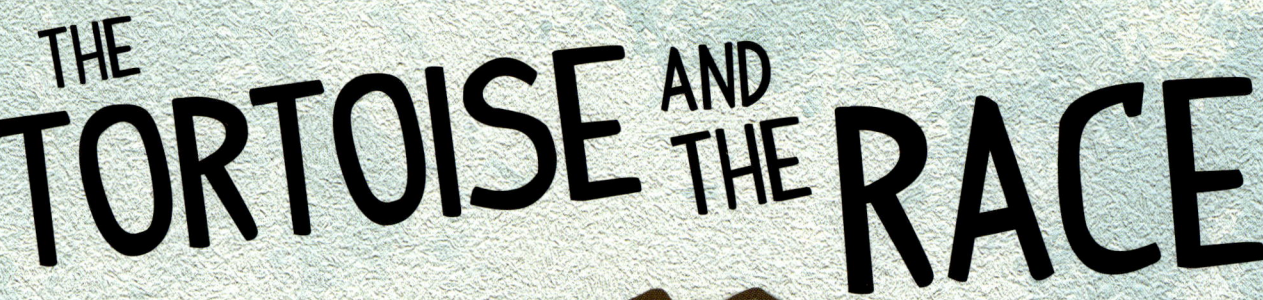

## THINK ABOUT IT

Stories can entertain us and inspire us. They can also educate us. Talk about a story that has taught you something.

**FOLK TALES ARE** stories that have been passed down from generation to generation. Many folk tales include animal characters that are a lot like humans. Most folk tales also include a moral or lesson. In this folk tale, Antelope and Tortoise organize a race to decide who is the older and wiser animal. Read on to see what happens.

One day, Tortoise decided he was in the mood for an adventure. He decided to leave his family for a little while and go on an excursion. On his way, he came upon the village where his friend Antelope lived. When Antelope saw Tortoise, Antelope insisted that Tortoise stay for dinner.

As they ate, the two friends had a lively conversation. They talked about many things. One thing they talked about was which one of them was older.

"I am older!" said Tortoise.

"No, I am older!" said Antelope.

In order to solve the disagreement, Tortoise suggested a race. The two of them would race each other. The winner would be considered the older of the two, and therefore the wiser. Antelope thought this was a good idea, so he agreed.

moral: *lesson about right and wrong*
excursion: *outing or short trip*

"I will surely be the winner!" laughed Antelope. "I can leap on my long legs. Tortoise crawls on his short legs!" Tortoise and Antelope decided the race would take place three days later.

Tortoise believed that preparing for this race was an adventure in itself. He returned home to his village. He sent word to all the other tortoises that he wanted to have a meeting with them. At the meeting, Tortoise told his friends and family that he had challenged Antelope to a very important race. However, he knew that Antelope was much faster than he was. He needed help from his friends in order to win.

Tortoise showed his friends where they would be racing, and he explained his plan. All the tortoises agreed to help out.

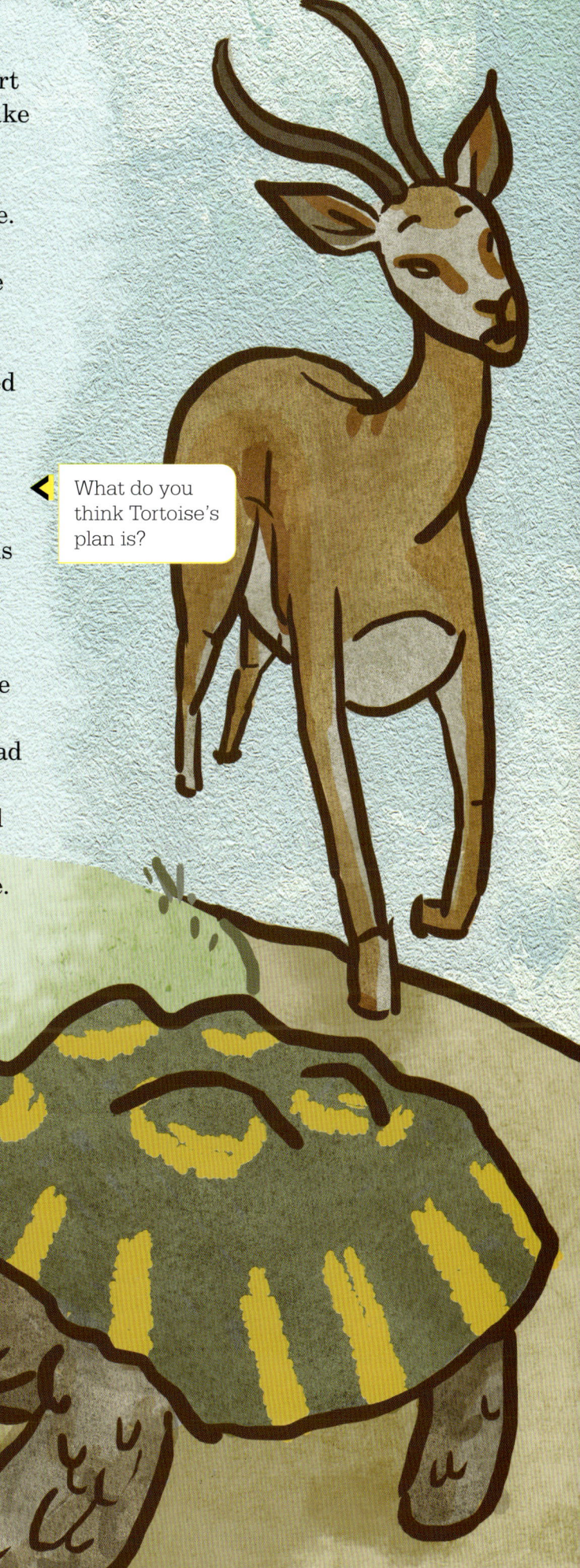

What do you think Tortoise's plan is?

The morning of the race came, and Tortoise and his friends got into their positions.

The race began, and Antelope took a big lead. As he approached the first village, he looked over his shoulder. He couldn't see Tortoise. He was sure that he had completely lost Tortoise. When he looked forward, however, he was shocked to see that Tortoise was ahead of him! Antelope ran even faster.

As Antelope approached the next village, he looked behind him again. Tortoise was nowhere to be seen. This time, Antelope knew he must be beating Tortoise. He was running so fast! And Tortoise was slow. As Antelope ran around a corner, he smiled to himself. But his smile quickly disappeared. Tortoise was running far ahead of him!

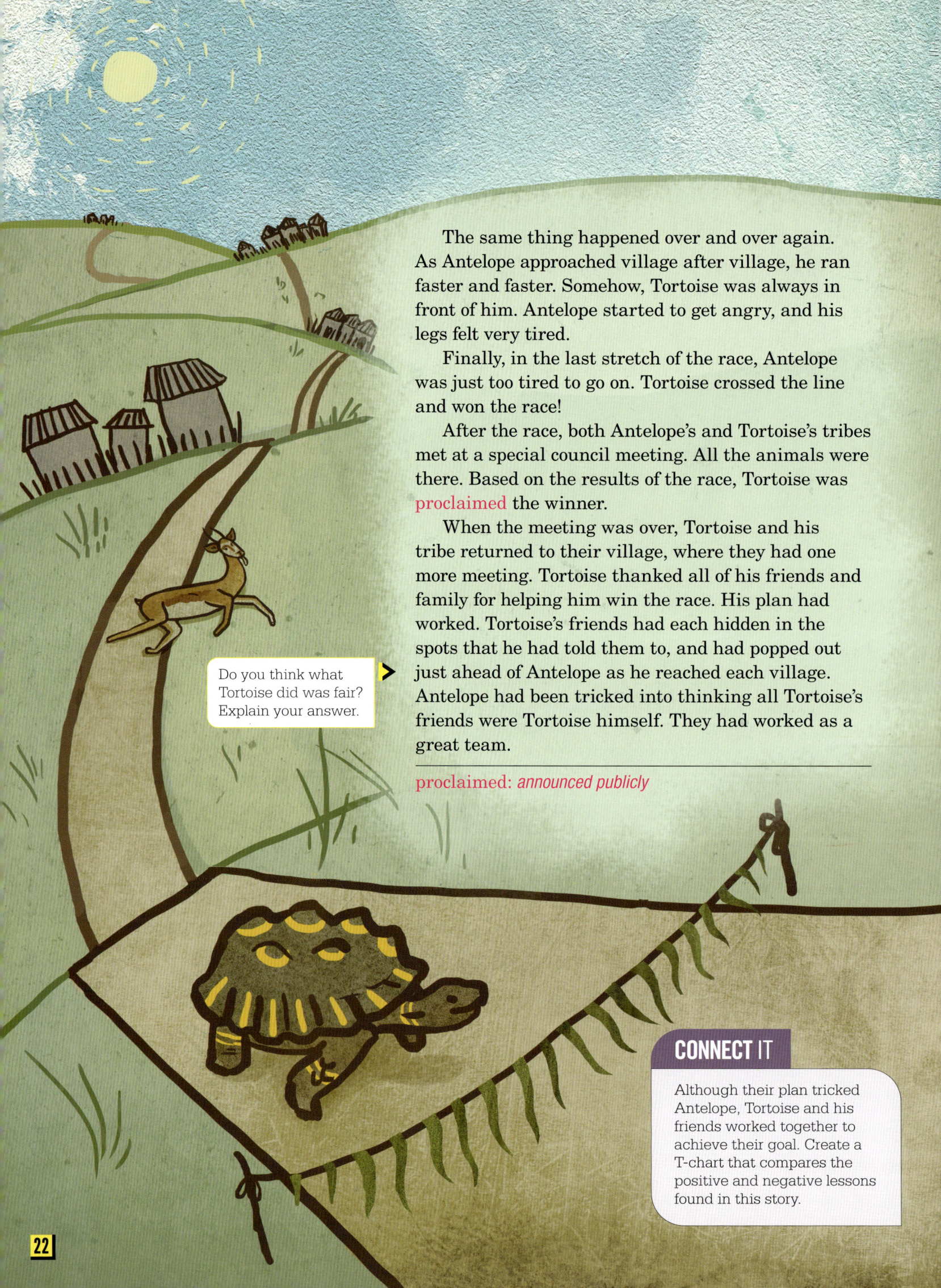

The same thing happened over and over again. As Antelope approached village after village, he ran faster and faster. Somehow, Tortoise was always in front of him. Antelope started to get angry, and his legs felt very tired.

Finally, in the last stretch of the race, Antelope was just too tired to go on. Tortoise crossed the line and won the race!

After the race, both Antelope's and Tortoise's tribes met at a special council meeting. All the animals were there. Based on the results of the race, Tortoise was proclaimed the winner.

When the meeting was over, Tortoise and his tribe returned to their village, where they had one more meeting. Tortoise thanked all of his friends and family for helping him win the race. His plan had worked. Tortoise's friends had each hidden in the spots that he had told them to, and had popped out just ahead of Antelope as he reached each village. Antelope had been tricked into thinking all Tortoise's friends were Tortoise himself. They had worked as a great team.

proclaimed: *announced publicly*

Do you think what Tortoise did was fair? Explain your answer.

**CONNECT IT**

Although their plan tricked Antelope, Tortoise and his friends worked together to achieve their goal. Create a T-chart that compares the positive and negative lessons found in this story.

# KEEPING FOLK TALES ALIVE

## THINK ABOUT IT

Think about an educational video game that you like to play. Share what you like about it with a partner.

**THE TORTOISE AND THE RACE** is just one of many folk tales that have been passed from generation to generation. Today, African game developers are preserving folk tales in a new way.

Folk tales are usually passed down orally from generation to generation. But that's not the only way to keep a story alive. Leti Games is incorporating traditional African folk tales into video games. Leti Games was created by Eryam Tawia and Wesley Kirinya. It is based in Ghana and Nigeria. Both Tawia and Kirinya have always loved playing video games. Yet they wondered why there were rarely Black characters featured in them. They decided to create their own games.

Tawia and Kirinya call themselves "technical geeks." They do a lot of the designing and programming of the games themselves. Their goal is to bring the rich folklore of Africa to life using mobile games and digital comics. Their mission is to bring African superheroes to the world.

One of their games, *Ananse: The Origin*, features the West African character Ananse. Ananse is a wise storyteller and a trickster. He is typically seen as a spider. However, in this game, Ananse takes on a human body, complete with incredible superpowers. Tawia and Kirinya say the game incorporates a lot of African mythology, themes, and culture. Tawia and Kirinya believe that a video game is the perfect way to share traditional African folk tales with a younger generation.

folklore: *traditional stories, beliefs, and customs*

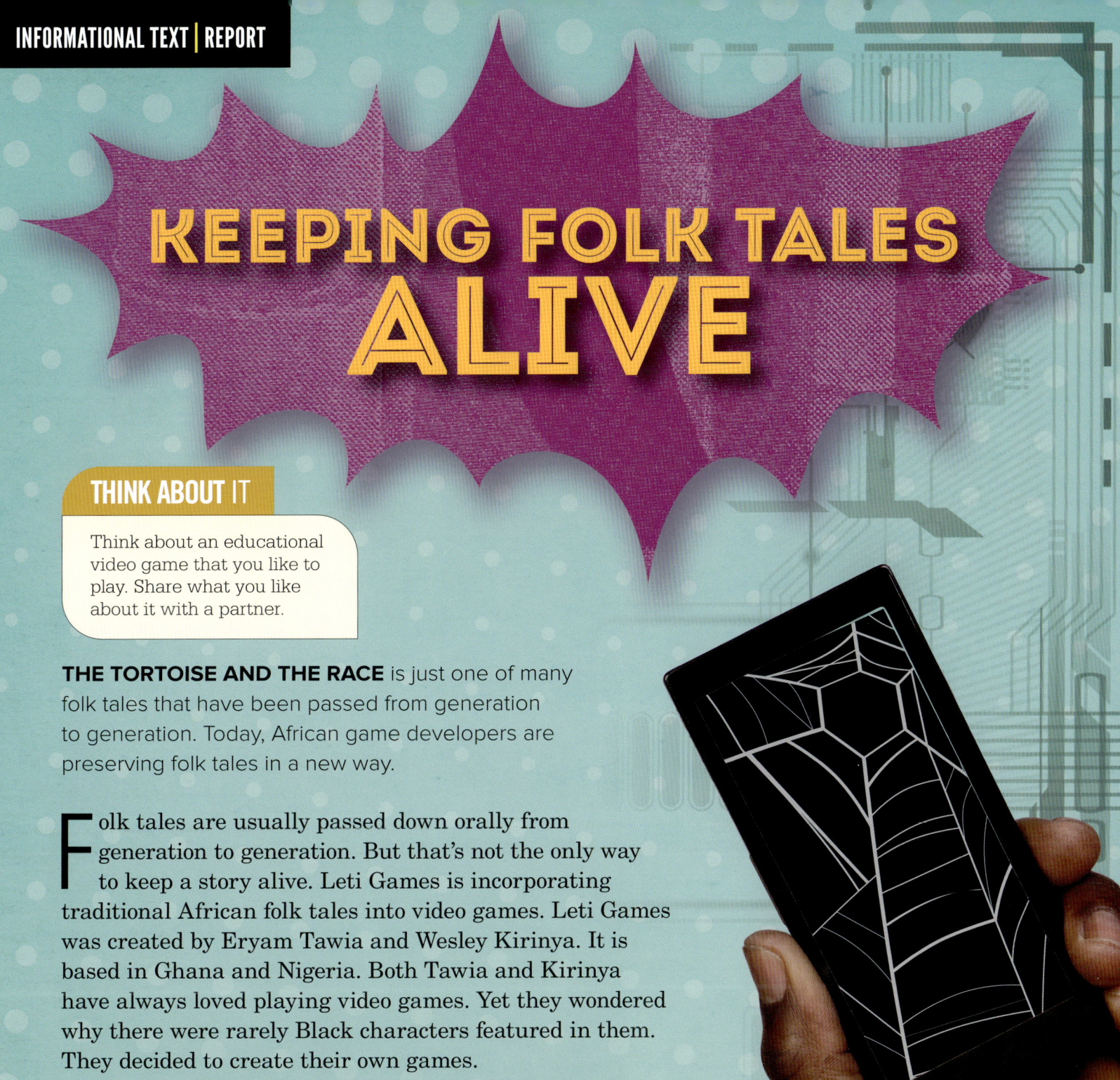

## CONNECT IT

Choose a traditional African folk tale. If you do not know one, do some research to find one. Write a short summary of the folk tale. How could it be turned into a video game?

# All About GAMES

**THE UNITED NATIONS** believes that all children in the world have the right to play. Life skills, such as teamwork, co-operation, and leadership, can be developed by playing games. There are many different reasons to play games. They entertain us. They keep our minds and bodies healthy. Games teach us how to think strategically and work as a team. They help us build our problem-solving skills and creativity. Read all about games in these fact cards.

"When children play, the world wins."

— International organization Right To Play

## Types of Games

According to the University of Waterloo, there are three basic types of games: racing, oppositional, and positional.

### Racing Games

The main goal of games in this category is to accomplish a certain task or arrive at a specific destination (the finish line, for example) before your opponent does.

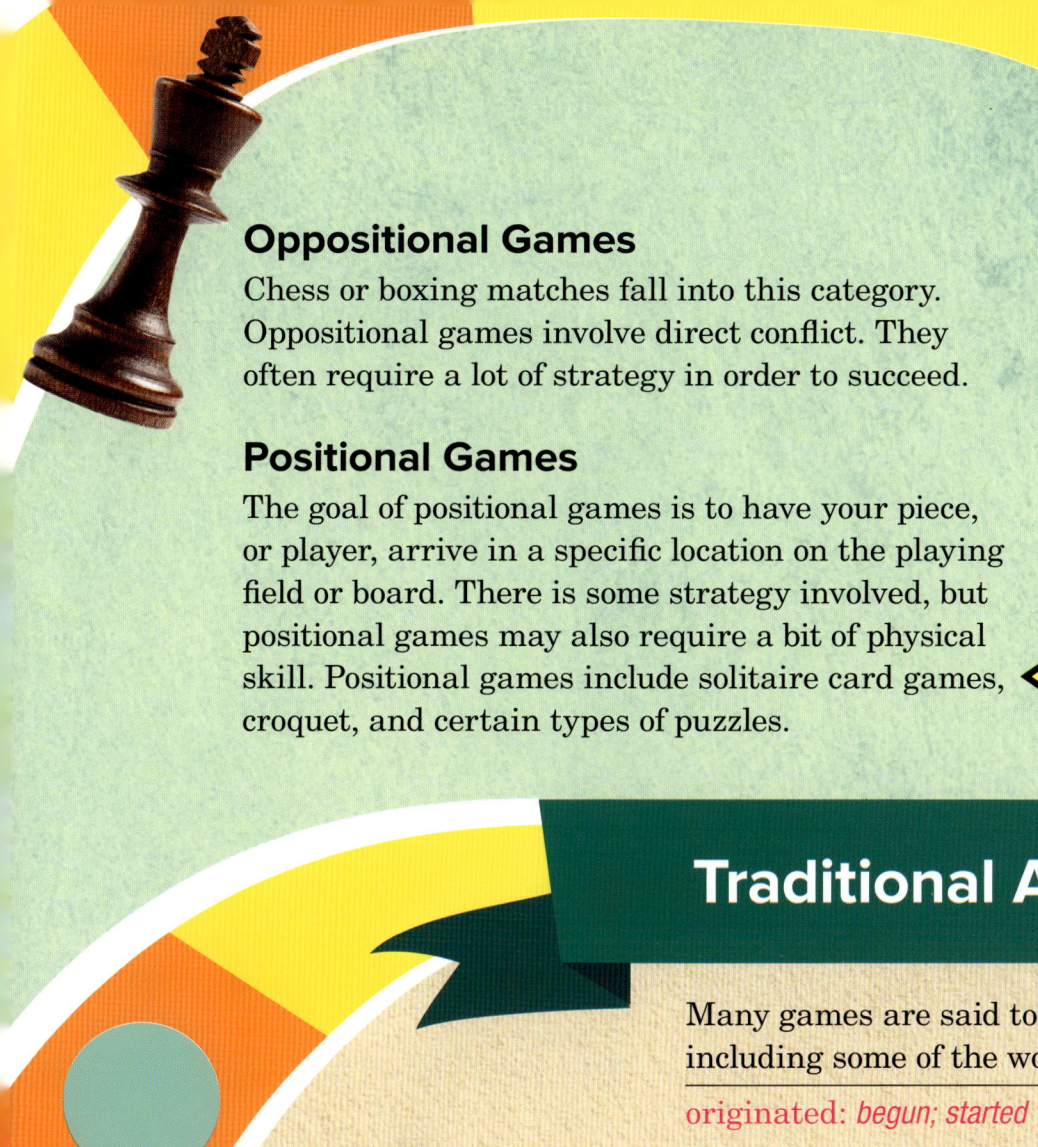

## Oppositional Games

Chess or boxing matches fall into this category. Oppositional games involve direct conflict. They often require a lot of strategy in order to succeed.

## Positional Games

The goal of positional games is to have your piece, or player, arrive in a specific location on the playing field or board. There is some strategy involved, but positional games may also require a bit of physical skill. Positional games include solitaire card games, croquet, and certain types of puzzles.

Can you think of any games that would fall under all three of these headings?

# Traditional African Games

Many games are said to have originated in Africa, including some of the world's oldest games.

originated: *begun; started*

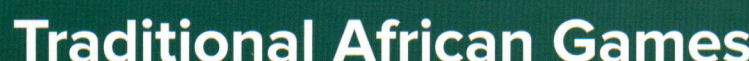

## Senet

Senet, a type of board game, is believed to have been played in Egypt as far back as 3500 BCE. Unfortunately, the rules to the game have been lost over the years. However, one thing is certain: Senet must have been very popular. Senet boards have been found etched onto ancient Egyptian tombs and hidden in burial chambers.

## Mancala

Mancala is another board game that dates back thousands of years. The word "mancala" is a common Arabic word. It means "to transfer." Originating in Africa, this game has also been called Wari. This game is played by moving stones strategically from one spot on the game board to another. It doesn't require expensive equipment. People in Malawi often scratch holes in the dirt to use as a board. They use pebbles as their pieces. This ancient game is still very popular today. You can even buy a Mancala board game at your local game store.

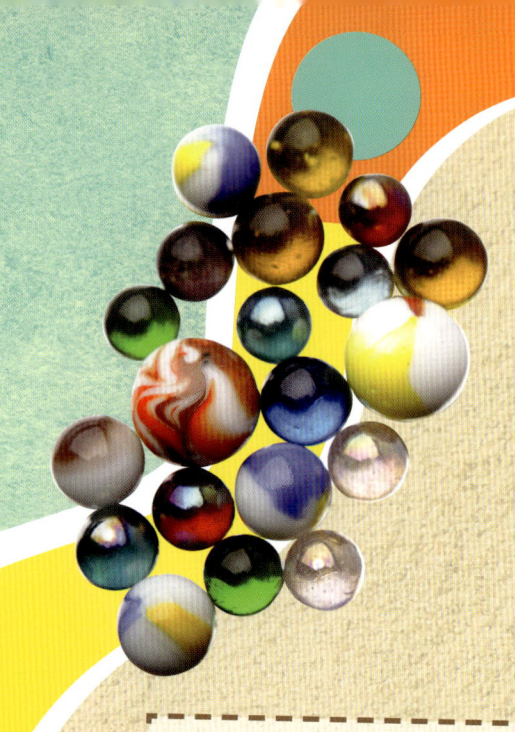

## Kudoda

This game is played mostly in Zimbabwe. Variations of it have been played all over the world. To play Kudoda, you need at least three players who sit in a circle around a bowl filled with 20 small stones or marbles. This game requires fast fingers. The first player throws a stone into the air, and then tries to pick up as many stones from the bowl as possible before the first stone drops to the ground. Each player gets a turn. At the end of the game, the person with the most stones wins.

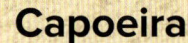

Variations: *different types*

## Nyama, Nyama

This Kenyan children's game has been compared to the Western game of "Simon Says." One person sits in the middle of a circle of children and says the name of an animal. The children jump up and yell "nyama" (which is Swahili for the word "meat") if that animal is eaten for food. If it isn't a type of food, the children will freeze, and make no sound at all. If a child gets excited and jumps up when the wrong animal is called out, the child goes into the centre of the circle, and the game begins again.

## Capoeira

Capoeira is a fascinating mix of martial arts, acrobatics, and dance. While it doesn't have a clear winner and loser, it is often thought of as a type of game. It is believed to have been invented hundreds of years ago in Brazil. Some people think it was used by enslaved Africans as a way to defend themselves, as well as keep parts of their culture alive. Practising capoeira was illegal until the early 1930s. Capoeira games take place in a large circle, known as a roda, and music sets the pace of the competition.

# Modern African Games

Traditional African games are moving into the 21st century. *MRBRB* is a digital game that was developed by a young South African university student. Based on a game played by cow herders in southern Africa called Morabaraba, the video game version, *MRBRB*, requires a great deal of strategy. The goal of the game is to build "mills" in order to capture your opponent's pieces, called "cows." People can play the game on a computer or smartphone.

There are hundreds of amazing video games out there that are not only fun to play but also teach us something. *Raiders of the Lost Bark*, developed by the Rainforest Foundation, helps to raise awareness about the destruction of the Congo. Wii even has a game called *Wild Earth: African Safari*, where players trek through the safari taking pictures of wildlife and observing the animals in their natural habitats.

The first Black video game character appeared in the Atari game *Basketball* in 1979. What other Black video game characters can you think of?

Video games can teach you to:
- think critically
- work hard to achieve a goal
- make decisions and solve problems
- collaborate with others
- handle failure

## CONNECT IT

Many children in Canada and around the world do not have access to store-bought toys or games. If you had only your imagination and a few pebbles, a tin can, a block of wood, and a piece of string, what type of game could you create? Write out the rules, and come up with a name for your new game.

# "Words of WISDOM"

## THINK ABOUT IT

What advice would you give to a friend who has encountered a challenge? Are there any inspirational sayings you would share with him or her?

**THE FOLLOWING INCREDIBLE** athletes share some inspirational advice about how to achieve your dreams.

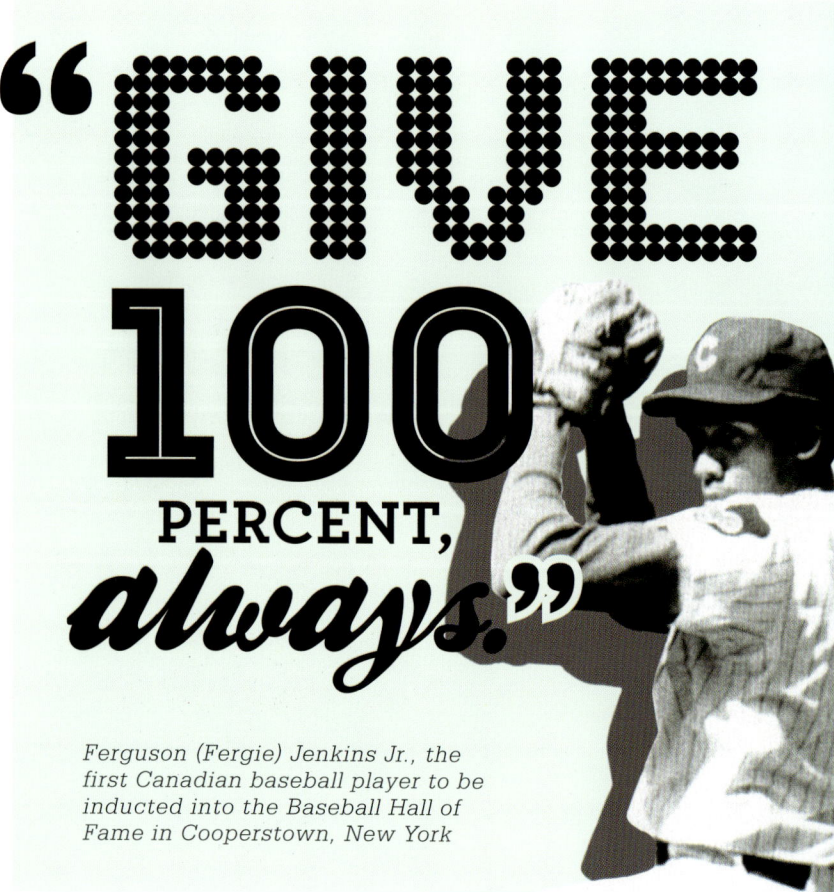

"GIVE 100 PERCENT, *always.*"

Ferguson (Fergie) Jenkins Jr., the first Canadian baseball player to be inducted into the Baseball Hall of Fame in Cooperstown, New York

"I'VE MISSED MORE THAN **9000** SHOTS IN MY CAREER. I'VE LOST ALMOST **300** games. I'VE FAILED OVER & OVER AGAIN IN MY LIFE. AND THAT IS WHY I SUCCEED."

Michael Jordan, American basketball superstar

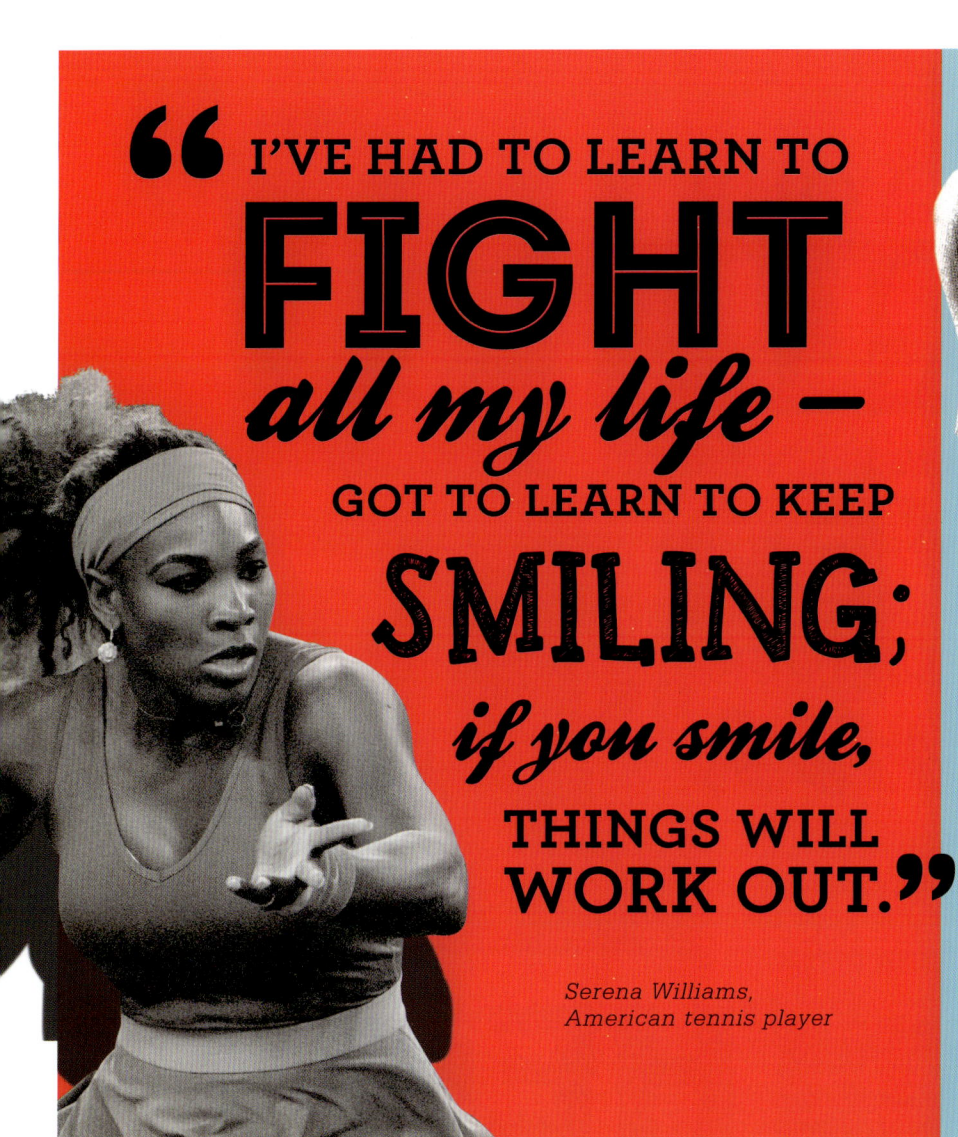

"I'VE HAD TO LEARN TO **FIGHT** *all my life –* GOT TO LEARN TO KEEP **SMILING;** *if you smile,* THINGS WILL WORK OUT."

*Serena Williams,*
*American tennis player*

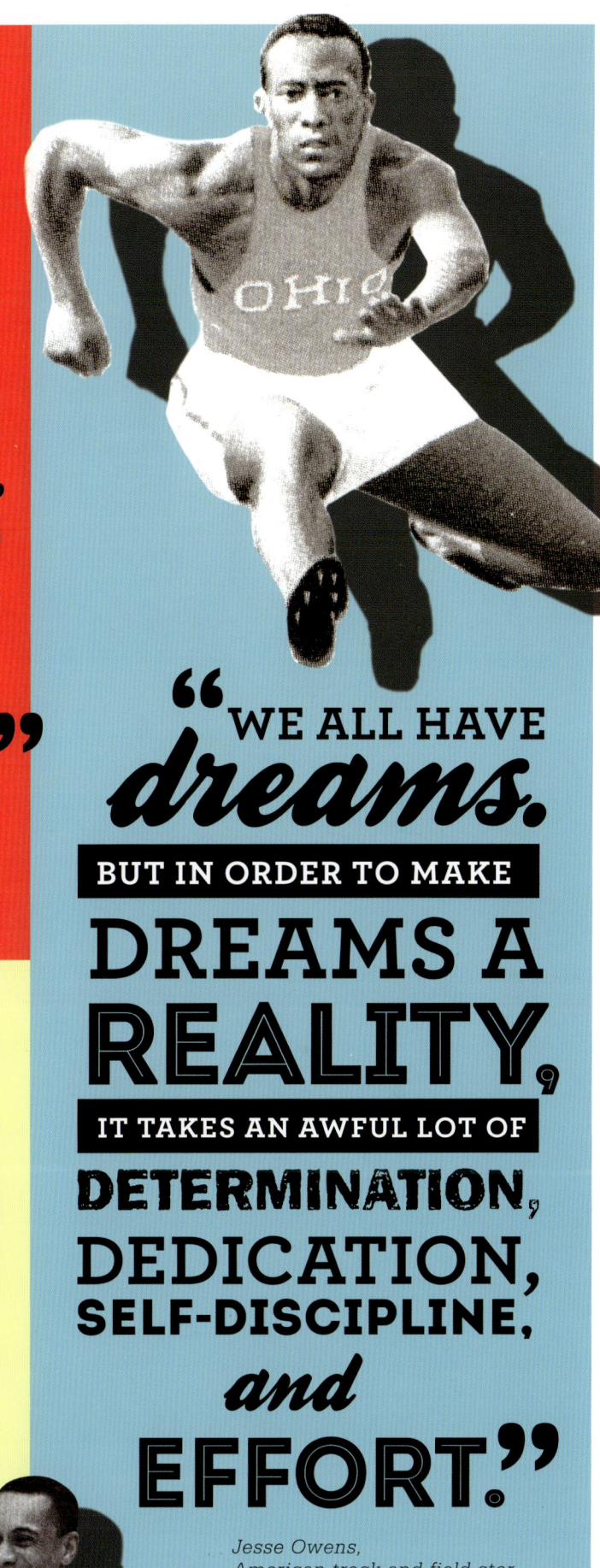

"WE ALL HAVE *dreams.* BUT IN ORDER TO MAKE DREAMS A REALITY, IT TAKES AN AWFUL LOT OF DETERMINATION, DEDICATION, SELF-DISCIPLINE, *and* EFFORT."

*Jesse Owens,*
*American track and field star*

"IF YOU SAY YOU CAN, THEN YOU CAN. IF YOU SAY *you can't,* THEN YOU ARE RIGHT."

*Willie O'Ree,*
*Canadian hockey player*

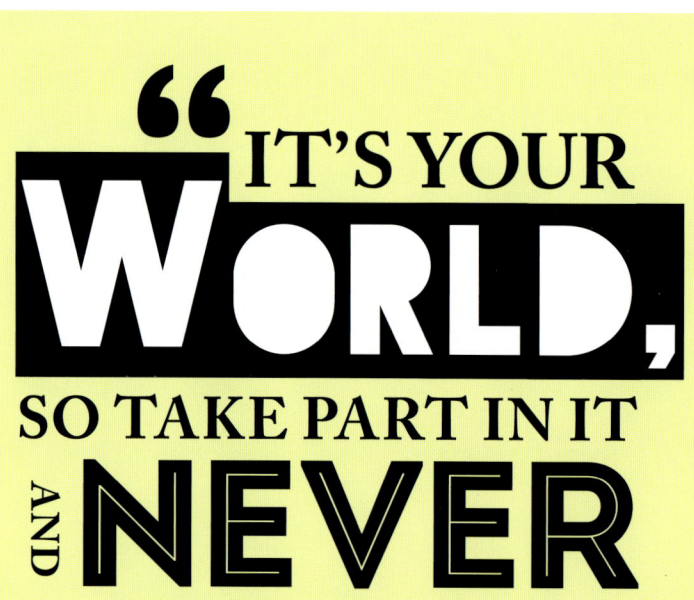

"IT'S YOUR **WORLD,** SO TAKE PART IN IT AND **NEVER** GIVE UP ON YOUR *dreams.*"

*Charmaine Crooks,*
*five-time Canadian Olympian*

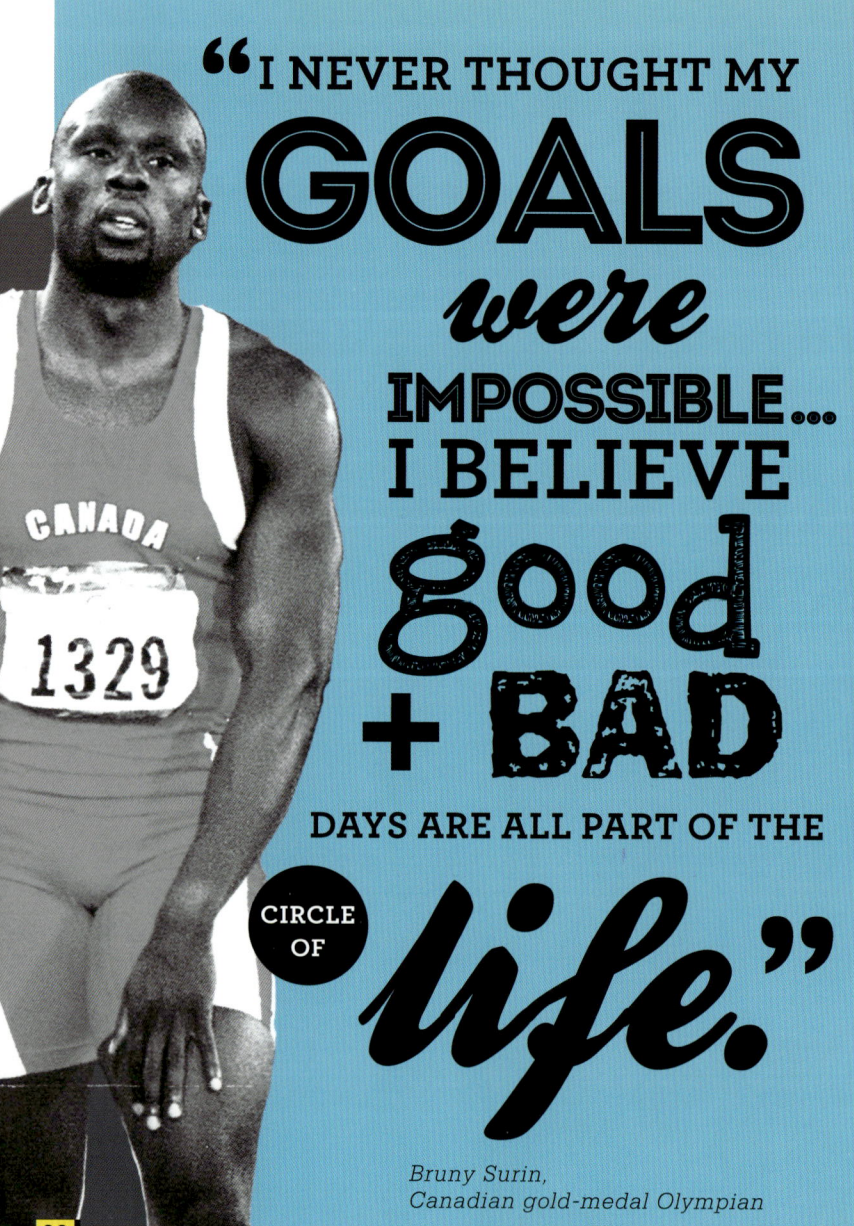

"I NEVER THOUGHT MY **GOALS** *were* IMPOSSIBLE... I BELIEVE *good* + **BAD** DAYS ARE ALL PART OF THE CIRCLE OF *life.*"

*Bruny Surin,*
*Canadian gold-medal Olympian*

"**HE** WHO IS **NOT** COURAGEOUS ENOUGH TO TAKE **RISKS** WILL ACCOMPLISH **NOTHING IN LIFE**"

*Muhammad Ali, American*
*heavyweight boxing champion*

**CONNECT** IT

Reread the quotations. Choose the ones that you think will be most helpful to you in your life. Explain your choices to a partner.

# Spotlight on Perdita Felicien

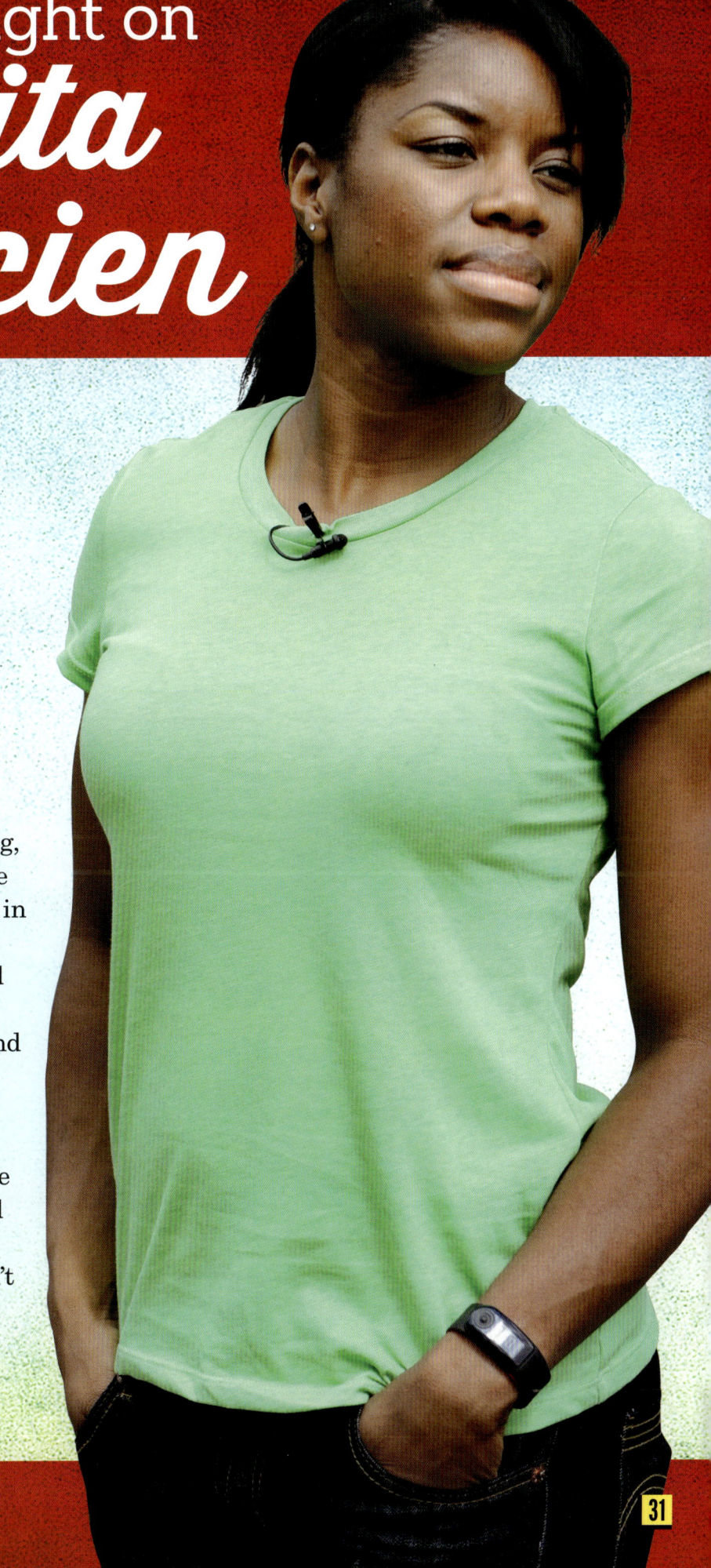

## THINK ABOUT IT

With a partner, talk about an obstacle you once had to overcome in order to do something that you wanted to do.

**WHAT DOES IT TAKE** to become an international track star? Read this profile of Perdita Felicien to find out.

Perdita Felicien was born in Oshawa, Ontario, in 1980. Her parents, three sisters, and brother moved to Pickering, Ontario, when Felicien was seven. In grade three, Felicien won an award of excellence in the Canada Fitness Award Program. That year, her teacher, Mrs. Arthur, encouraged her to try out for the track and field team. She started competing in the 100-metre and 200-metre dash, as well as long jump. At this time, she didn't like running hurdles.

Felicien won a lot of competitions while she was in elementary school. However, the thought of competing in high school scared her. She had become used to being one of the best. She was worried that she wouldn't be able to succeed if she competed on a high-school team, so she decided to quit track and field.

Felicien's mother was worried that her daughter was wasting her talent. Much to Felicien's annoyance, her mother kept encouraging her to go back to track and field. All this prodding made her even more reluctant to return to the track.

Finally, at the age of 14, Felicien decided to give track and field another try. Surprisingly, it was the hurdles where she really excelled. Felicien went on to win a national junior title in hurdling. She broke provincial records and attracted the attention of scouts from American universities. She was offered an athletic scholarship from the University of Illinois when she was 19.

## This was the first time a Canadian woman had won a gold medal at the championships.

In university, Felicien worked incredibly hard. In her first year, she set a record in the 100-metre hurdles event. She ran faster than any freshman ever had in National Collegiate Athletic Association (NCAA) history. In 2003, she found herself competing in Paris, France, at the International Association of Athletics Federations (IAAF) World Championships. She won the 100-metre hurdles final. This was the first time a Canadian woman had won a gold medal at the championships.

In 2004, Felicien graduated from university with a Bachelor of Science degree in kinesiology. At the same time, she continued to experience great success in the hurdling world. She competed in the Summer Olympic Games in Athens, Greece. Many Canadians cheered while she ran the 100-metre final and gasped when she tripped over the first hurdle. Felicien didn't achieve her Olympic dream of winning a medal.

scouts: *people who travel around looking for exceptional athletes*
National Collegiate Athletic Association (NCAA): *organization in the United States that runs college and university athletic programs*
kinesiology: *study of how the human body moves*

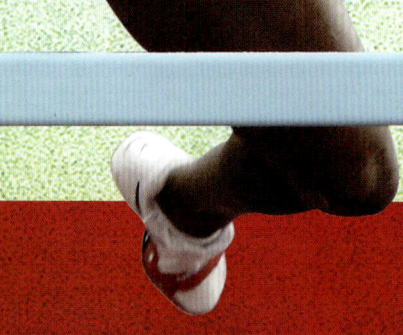

*Perdita Felicien competes at the 10th IAAF World Athletics Championships in Helsinki, Finland, on 10 August 2005.*

Felicien was crushed, but she picked herself up and moved on. She trained harder and ran faster, and went on to win a silver medal at another IAAF World Championships in 2007. Although she couldn't compete in the 2008 Beijing Olympics because of a foot injury, she did travel to Beijing. She was a guest commentator for CBC's coverage of the Olympic hurdle competitions. This was the beginning of her journalism career.

Felicien still dreamed of standing on an Olympic podium with a medal hanging around her neck. She spent the summer of 2011 training for the upcoming Olympics in London, England. However, Felicien made a false start in the Olympic trials, and was disqualified. She never competed in another Olympics.

After Felicien didn't make the 2012 Olympic team, she decided to go back to school. She studied journalism, and worked as a television reporter in Hamilton, Ontario. She is also an ambassador for Right To Play. Right To Play is an organization that uses the fun of sports and games to help children around the world who are facing adversity. Felicien helps the organization by travelling to schools to talk to students about the importance of fair play and being active. Felicien also supports Count Me In, an organization promoting student volunteerism. It is the largest organization in Canada that is run by youth.

ambassador: *someone who represents a company or organization and helps to spread its message*
adversity: *hardship; suffering*

*Perdita Felicien announces her retirement from sports in 2013.*

## CONNECT IT

Imagine you had the opportunity to interview Felicien. What questions would you ask her about her career as an athlete? What questions would you ask her about her career as a journalist? Consider the similarities and differences in these two careers.

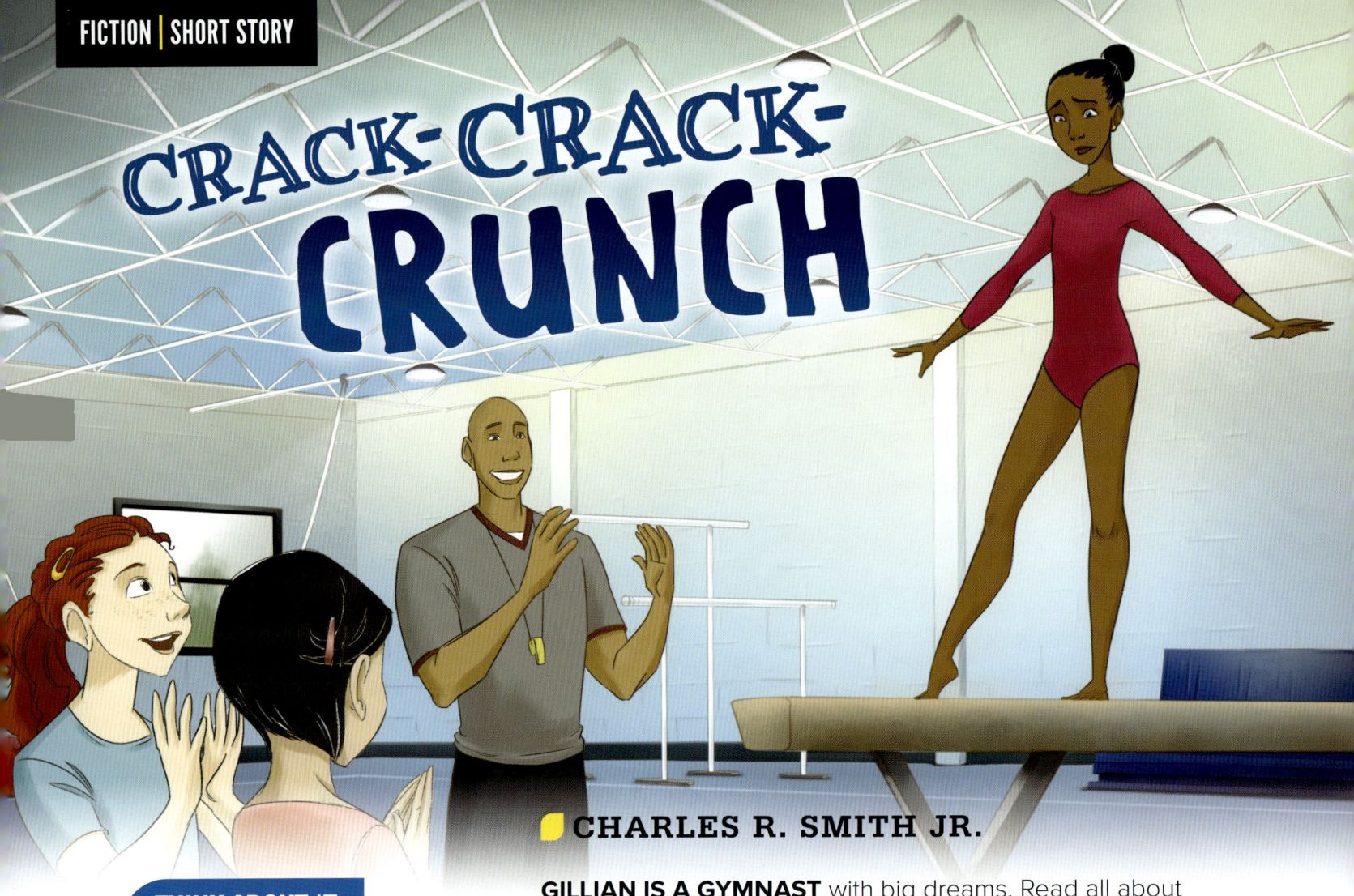

# CRACK-CRACK-CRUNCH

**CHARLES R. SMITH JR.**

**GILLIAN IS A GYMNAST** with big dreams. Read all about her in this short story by Charles R. Smith Jr.

## THINK ABOUT IT

Has there ever been a time when you did not believe in yourself? What did you do about this feeling? Write down your thoughts.

## ABOUT THE AUTHOR

Charles R. Smith Jr. is an American author, illustrator, and photographer. He is also a huge sports fan. Many of his children's books and poems are about sports.

"Come on, Gillian, let's see that back handspring! You did it on the floor no problem. You did it on the low beam no problem. Now let's see it on the high beam!"

Four inches wide. Four feet high. Sixteen feet long. The balance beam. The sixteen feet long I have no problem with; it's the four-feet-high and four-inches-wide part that worries me. So far, it's been easy because we've been doing stuff forward, but now we have to learn to go backward to move to the next level.

Every time I get up here, I have to calm myself down and relax. My heart starts racing and leaps up into my throat. My palms get sweaty. My head starts throbbing. My vision gets blurry when I look down. My calf muscles start twitching, and I get chicken skin everywhere. I try, but I never relax. I always feel like I'm going to break a bone. Or two. Or ten.

"Come on, Gillian, let's go!"

Let's go. The two words Coach always uses to kick me into gear. The two words that mean it's time to say goodbye to another fear. I mean, that's all gymnastics is really about: fear. Fear of not doing something right. Fear of embarrassing yourself. Fear of breaking something.

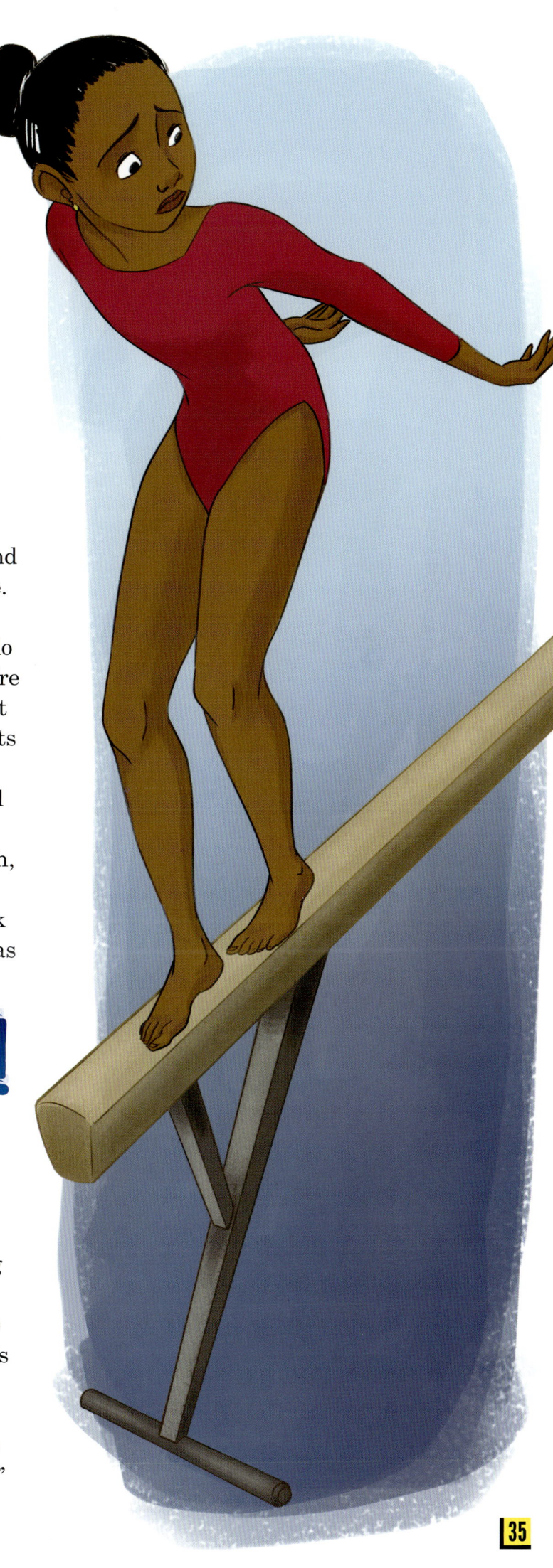

My first-ever backflip years ago was kind of freaky because my body had never done that before. Once my feet left the ground, though … oh, man … it was like my body just knew what to do. Before I knew it, I was on my feet, and Coach was clapping up a storm and shouting, "Yeah!"

Coach is clapping again now — not for what I just did, but to help me do what I need to do.

"Come on, Gillian. Practice is almost over. It would be so awesome if you could end it on a high note. I know you can do it."

I can't do this. I need more practice. Maybe I can do it tomorrow. Or next week. Who am I kidding? I'm just not ready. I say this to Coach, and he just looks me in the eye and says, "Yes, you are. Let's go!"

I was one of the first ones in the class ever to do a backflip because I didn't care if I fell. When you're five years old, you don't think about that stuff. But now … it's a different story. Our team has done lots of meets and competed in lots of events, so we've all seen some pretty crazy stuff. I've seen girls fall off the beam and twist their ankles, break their wrists, and land on their heads. The worst, though, was seeing this one girl fall off the beam and try to break her fall with her arm. Well, she did break her fall. And her arm, too. I remember it like it was yesterday. Run–run–run; round-off; back fl — …

# Crack–Cr–Crack!

She started her flip, but her hands never touched the beam. Everything happened so fast, but when I heard that sound … that bone snapping — UGH … I told myself, I'm never doing one of those up there.

"All right, Gillian, the clock is ticking. If you're not going to try it, let me give one of the other girls a chance."

I tell Coach I want to practise on the floor, so I hop off. Before I can move over to a larger mat, he tells me, "You're still going to try it today, though."

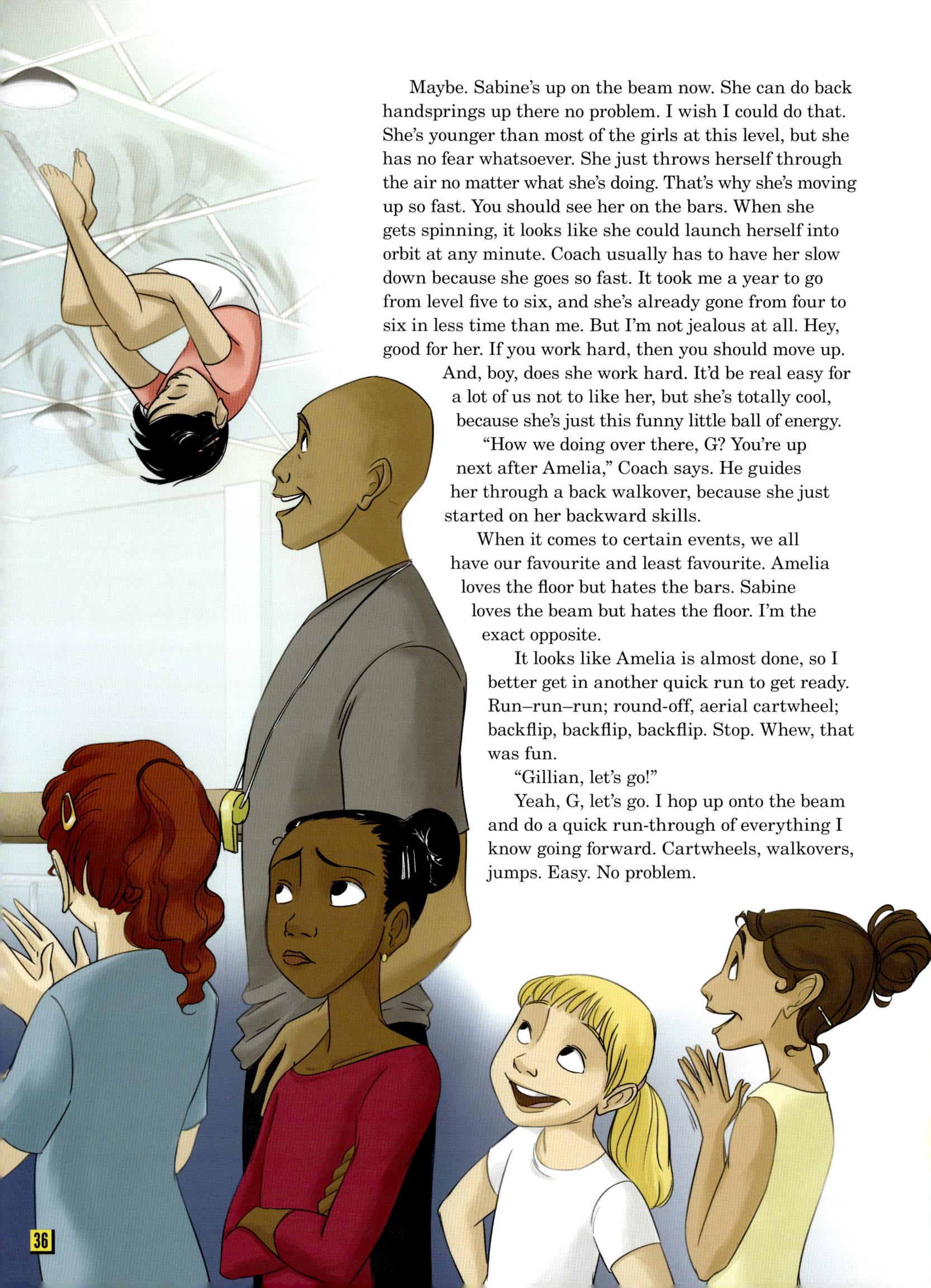

Maybe. Sabine's up on the beam now. She can do back handsprings up there no problem. I wish I could do that. She's younger than most of the girls at this level, but she has no fear whatsoever. She just throws herself through the air no matter what she's doing. That's why she's moving up so fast. You should see her on the bars. When she gets spinning, it looks like she could launch herself into orbit at any minute. Coach usually has to have her slow down because she goes so fast. It took me a year to go from level five to six, and she's already gone from four to six in less time than me. But I'm not jealous at all. Hey, good for her. If you work hard, then you should move up.

And, boy, does she work hard. It'd be real easy for a lot of us not to like her, but she's totally cool, because she's just this funny little ball of energy.

"How we doing over there, G? You're up next after Amelia," Coach says. He guides her through a back walkover, because she just started on her backward skills.

When it comes to certain events, we all have our favourite and least favourite. Amelia loves the floor but hates the bars. Sabine loves the beam but hates the floor. I'm the exact opposite.

It looks like Amelia is almost done, so I better get in another quick run to get ready. Run–run–run; round-off, aerial cartwheel; backflip, backflip, backflip. Stop. Whew, that was fun.

"Gillian, let's go!"

Yeah, G, let's go. I hop up onto the beam and do a quick run-through of everything I know going forward. Cartwheels, walkovers, jumps. Easy. No problem.

"All right, now let's see it backward," Coach says. He stands way off to the side, letting me know he isn't going to spot me. I stare down at the beam, and into my head pops a picture of bone poking out of flesh, while into my ears pops a loud —

# Crack–Cr–Crack!

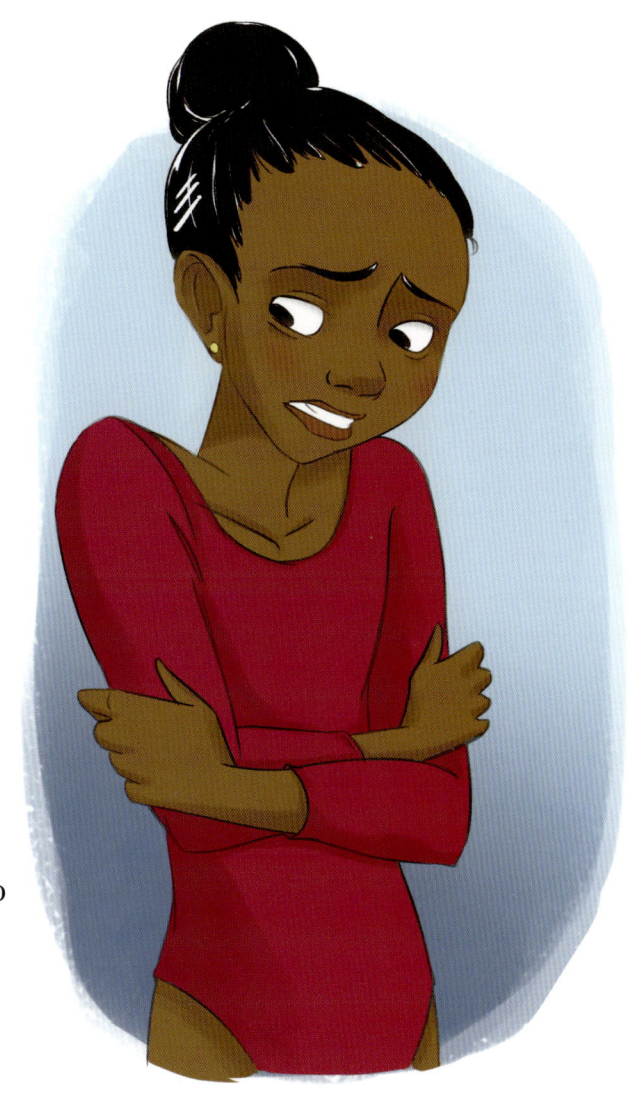

What if I fall? I can't see where my feet are gonna land … so what if I fall off and break my arm? Or something else? Coach can't say it won't happen, because I've seen it happen.

"I can't do this, Coach. What if I fall?"

"So you fall. It won't be the first time you've fallen, and it won't be the end of the world. If you don't at least try, then nothing will happen. Is that what you want? You've been making great progress so far. Do you want to stop right here, or do you wanna move up?"

Of course I wanna move up. I need to move up. I can do all the skills in the other events, so I need to move up. I can't let this hold me back. Come on, G. If little Sabine can do it, what do you have to be afraid of?

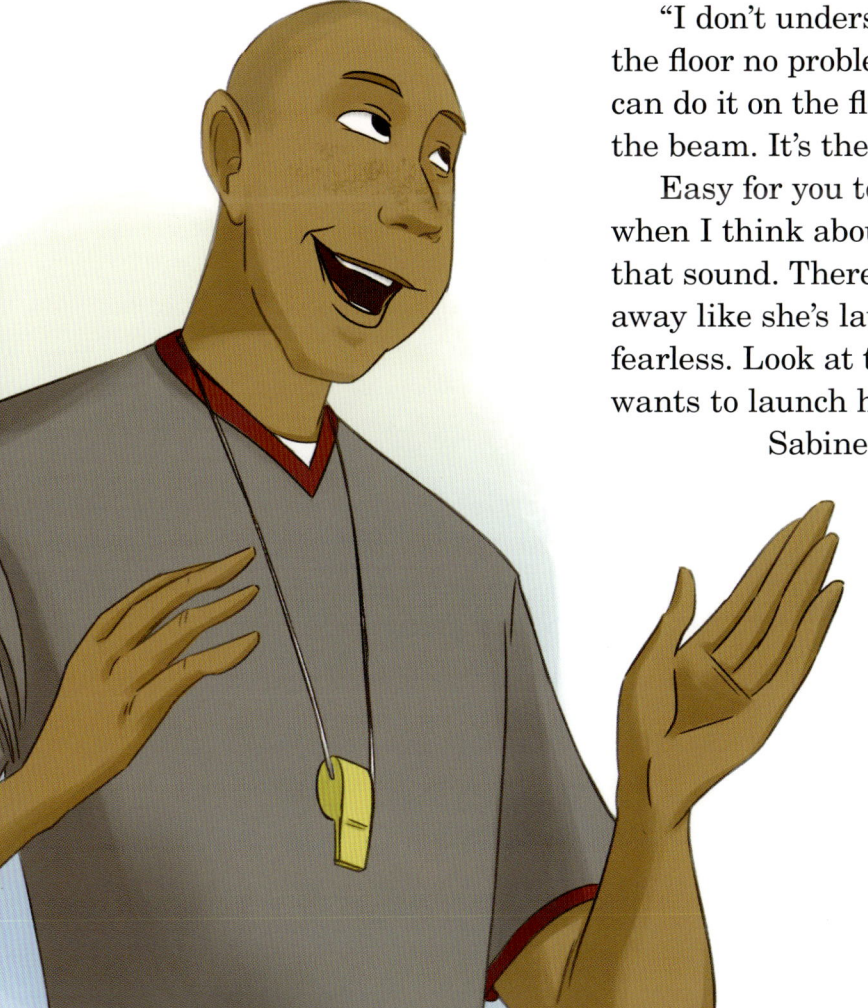

"I don't understand, Gillian. You do back handsprings on the floor no problem. I mean, you're one of the best. If you can do it on the floor in a straight line, then you can do it on the beam. It's the same thing. Just pretend it's the floor."

Easy for you to say, Coach. That's not what I think about when I think about the beam. All I can think about is … that sound. There goes Sabine on the uneven bars, swinging away like she's launching herself into space again. The girl's fearless. Look at that smile on her face. It looks like she wants to launch herself into space. Come on, Gillian. If little Sabine can do it, there's no reason you can't.

All right, let's give it a shot. Close your eyes. Pretend like you're on the floor. Don't think about being on the beam. Don't worry about falling —

Oh, man! As soon as I say don't think about it, of course I think about it.

Try something new. I need to get that sound out of my head. Every time I look at the beam, it echoes through my eardrums.

I lift my eyes off the beam and let them wander around the gym. Everyone has stopped. Some of the girls are hanging out on the mat, cheering me on. The rest are hovering around the snack bar. The popcorn machine is popping a fresh batch, and Sabine is wedging herself up front for a fresh bag.

The bags start filling, and soon Sabine and the other girls are on the mat, cheering me on between cracks and crunches of fresh popcorn.

"Come on, Gillian."

"Let's go!"

## Crack-Crack-Crunch!

Coach tells the girls to keep the noise down, but I say, "No, Coach, let 'em crunch as loud as they want."

The louder the better. I'd much rather hear popcorn crunching than — Come on, G. You can do this.

All right. Like Coach says, "LET'S GO!" Deep breaths. Arms up. Swing arms back. Arms behind head. Arch back. See the ceiling. Jump. Feet off the beam. Flip. Find the beam. See the beam. Hands on beam. Whip legs around. Keep feet straight. Whip feet over. Right foot, touch beam. Left foot, touch beam behind right foot. Stand. Arms up. Done. Smile.

Coach starts clapping, and the others join him.

"Great job, Gillian! I knew you could do it! How'd that feel?"

I hop off the beam and plunge my hand into Sabine's bag.

"Great! Now I'm hungry!"

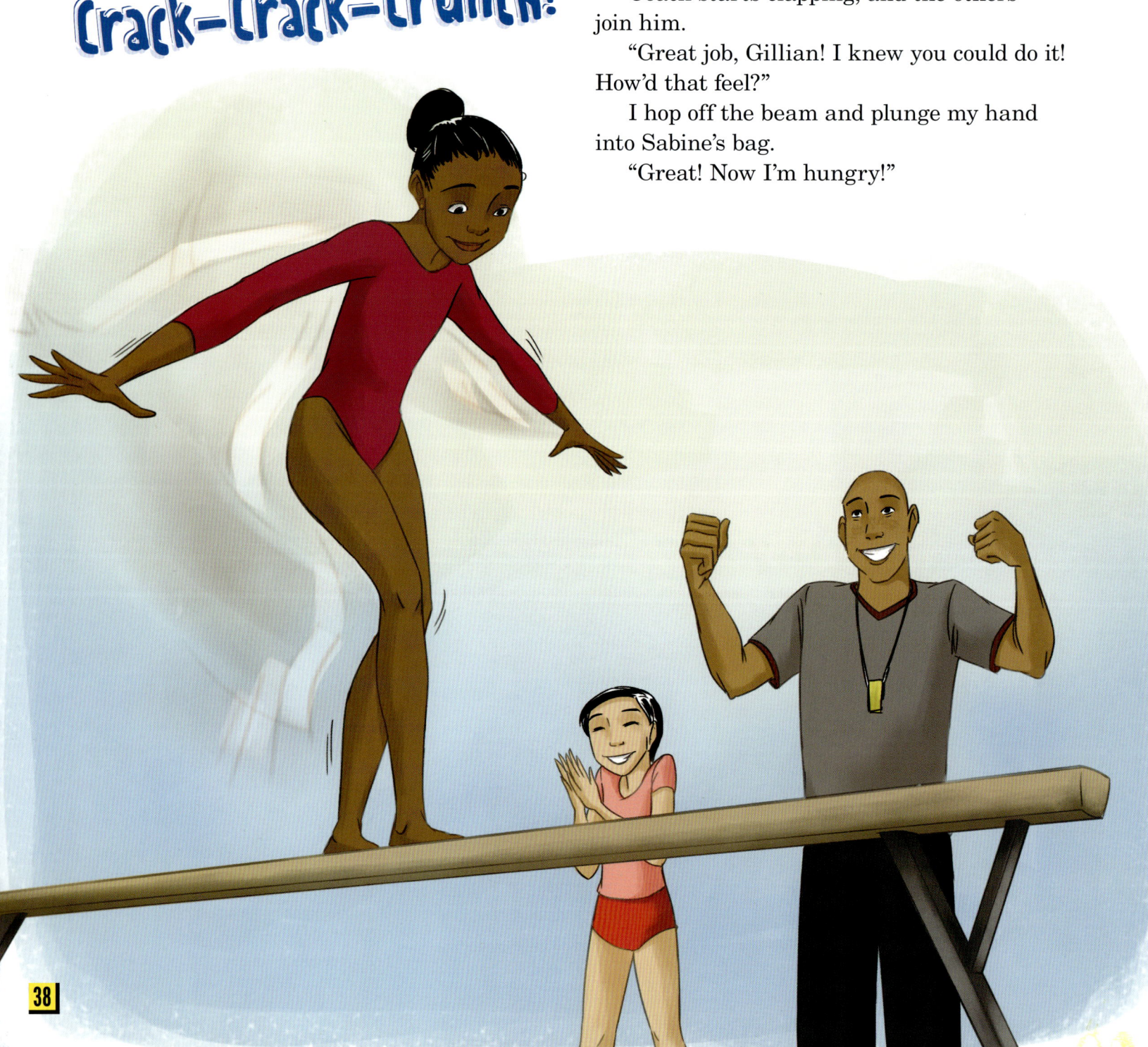

# A REAL-LIFE GYMNAST

Curtis Hibbert is a Canadian gymnast who competed in two Olympic Games. In the 1988 Olympic Games, he became the first Canadian gymnast to make the finals in three events. That year, in other competitions, he won 11 medals in international competitions. After his professional career ended, he created the Super Kids Gym Club, a non-competitive gymnastics centre that encouraged kids to get involved in gymnastics.

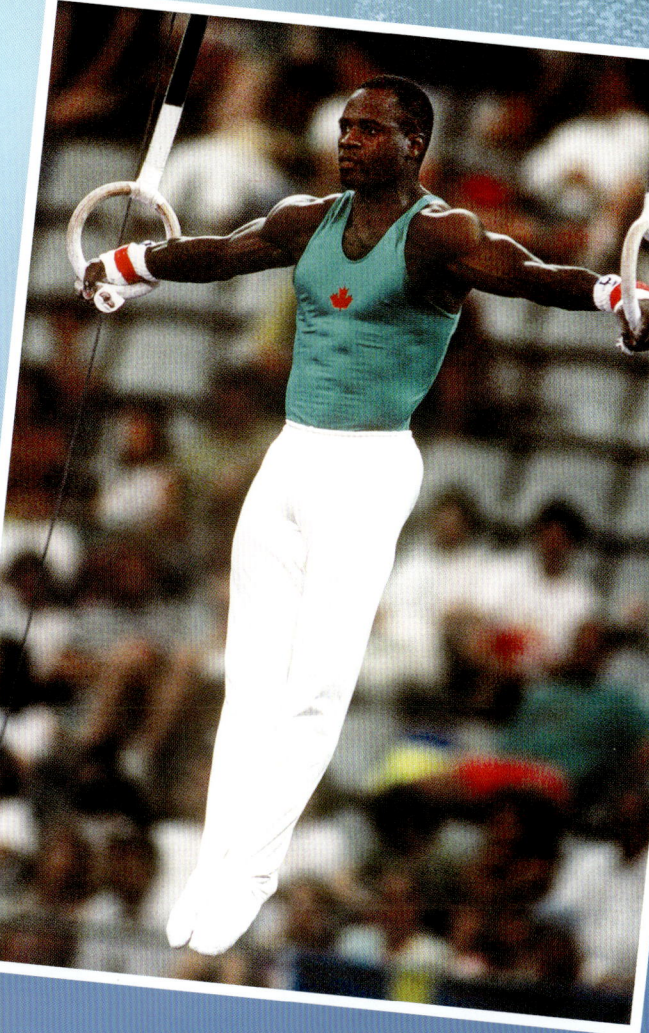

Hibbert competes in a ring event at the 1992 Olympic Games in Barcelona, Spain.

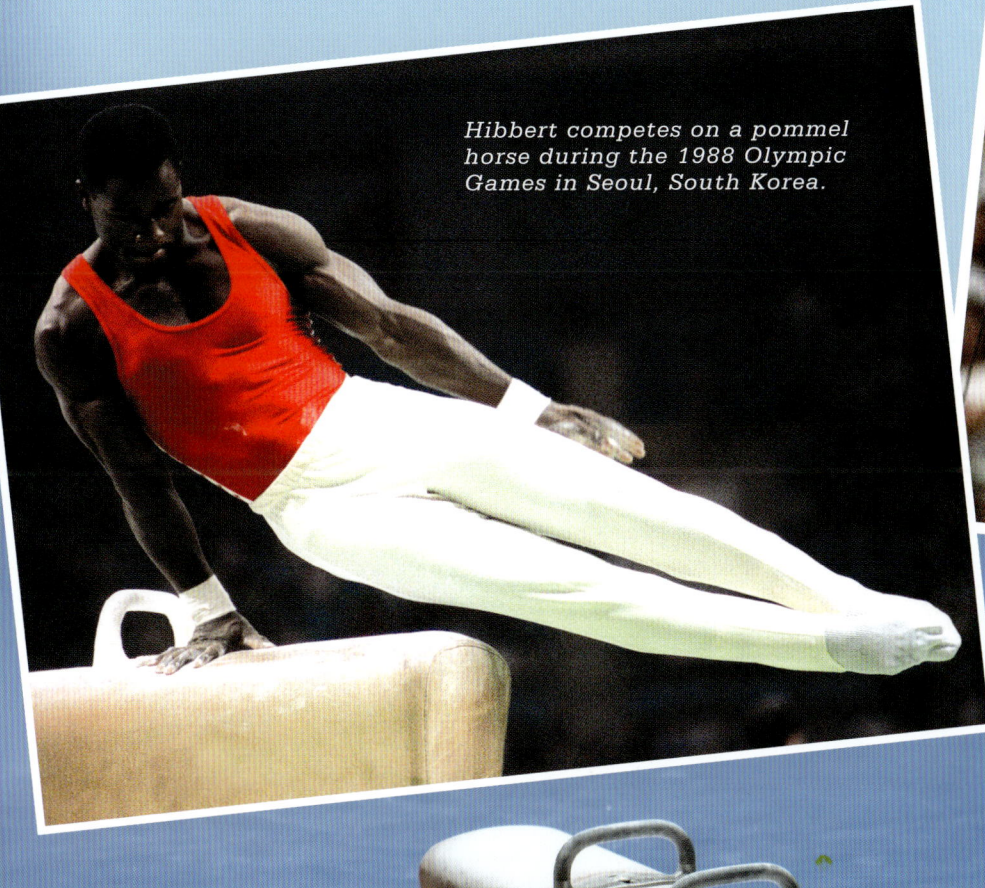

Hibbert competes on a pommel horse during the 1988 Olympic Games in Seoul, South Korea.

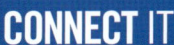

## CONNECT IT

In the voice of one of the characters in the story "Crack–Crack–Crunch," write a journal entry about the experience of competing in gymnastics. What emotions do you think a gymnast feels?

# SPORT
## HAS THE POWER
## TO CHANGE THE WORLD

**THINK ABOUT** IT

What role do sports play in your life? Share your thoughts with a partner.

**"SPORT HAS THE POWER** to change the world." These famous words were spoken by South African leader Nelson Mandela. "It has the power to inspire. It has the power to unite people in a way that little else does. It speaks to youth in a language they understand. Sport can create hope where once there was only despair."

Nelson Mandela knew a lot about changing the world. He spent his entire life working to end racism and Apartheid in South Africa. Mandela was the leader of a group that the government banned. He was put in jail for 27 years for challenging the government's system of Apartheid. Upon his release, he was still fiercely committed to unifying his country. One way he did this was through sport.

An amateur boxer and long-distance runner, Mandela stayed physically active while he was in prison. He spent 18 of his 27 years in prison on Robben Island. During his time there, the prisoners had formed a soccer league. Although Mandela wasn't allowed to join because he was in isolation, he secretly followed the games. According to Anthony Suze, a political prisoner during this time, "We played soccer on Robben Island with such passion and such detail — it was another way of survival. ... In a situation that sought to undermine us, it gave us hope."

In 1994, after Apartheid ended, Mandela became the first Black president of South Africa. The end of Apartheid meant many changes for the people of South Africa, though Black people were still not treated equally. There was still a lot of violence and suffering in the country.

Apartheid: *system in South Africa where White people controlled the country and decided where non-Whites could live, go to school, etc.*

For many years during Apartheid, South Africa had been banned from participating in international sporting events. This was because many other countries did not agree with Apartheid. Because of this, it was very important when South Africa hosted the Rugby World Cup in 1995. The Springboks, South Africa's rugby team, competed in the tournament.

In 1995, rugby was considered by many to be a White person's game. Most Springboks fans were White. Many Black South Africans viewed rugby as a reminder of the suffering they had experienced. By allowing the tournament to take place, Mandela was making a brave decision. Many people were worried that there would be violence. Mandela believed that the sporting event would help bring Black and White people in South Africa together.

When Mandela arrived at the stadium wearing a Springboks jersey, the team's captain couldn't believe it.

"I bit my lip so hard. I wanted to cry," said François Pienaar years later. Together, Black and White South Africans cheered for the national team. South Africa went on to win the entire tournament. Citizens of all races and ethnicities celebrated the win together. As Mandela said, "Sport has the power to change the world."

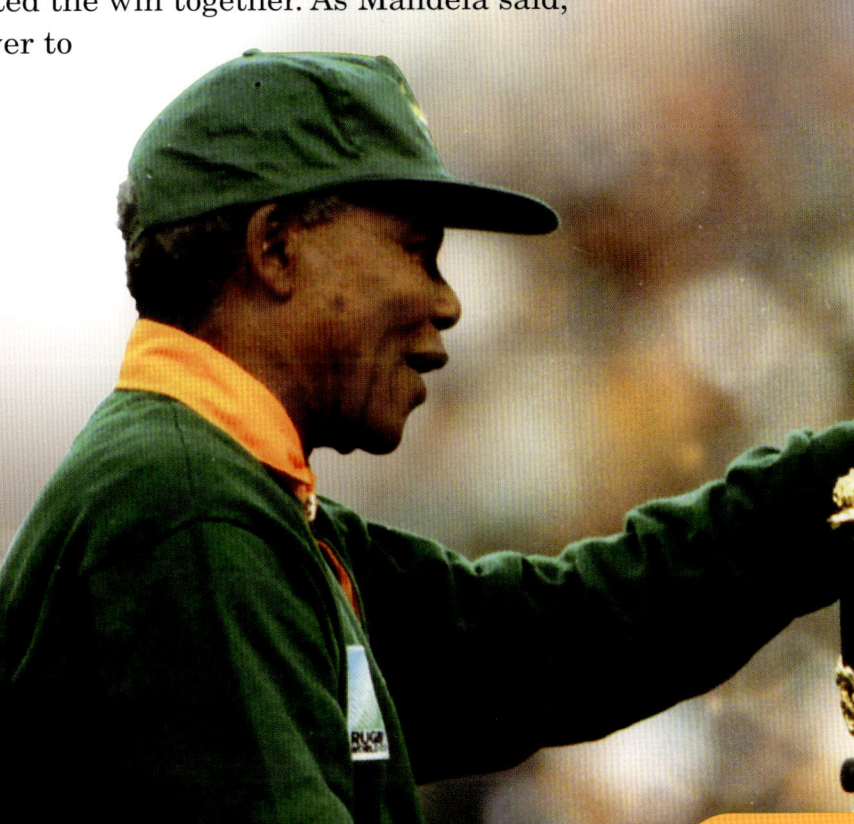

*Mandela congratulates Springboks captain François Pienaar on winning the 1995 Rugby World Cup.*

## CONNECT IT

Use the Web and other resources to find another example of sports being a powerful tool for change. Write a paragraph about this event that could be added to this opinion piece.

# Making the World a

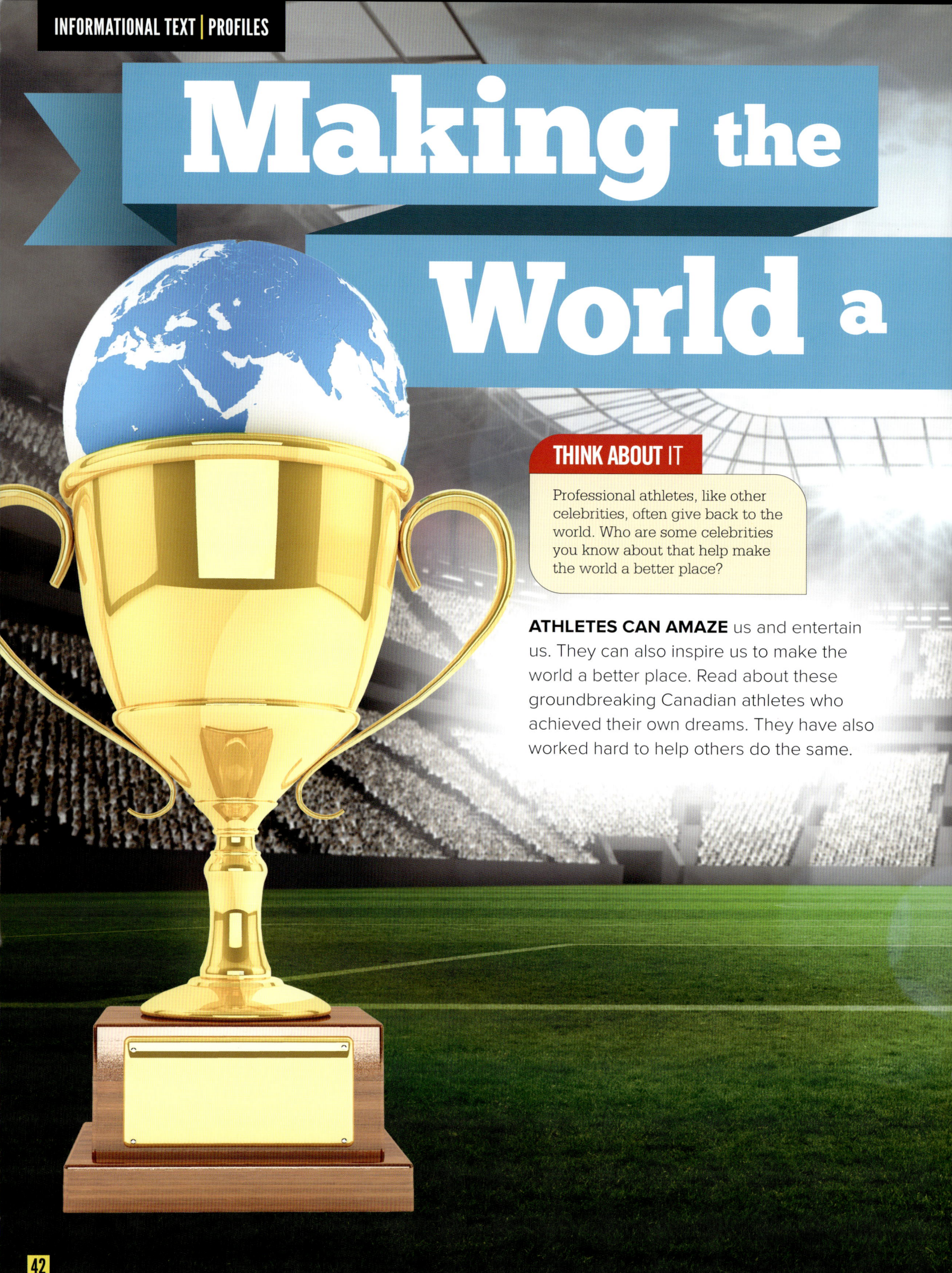

**ATHLETES CAN AMAZE** us and entertain us. They can also inspire us to make the world a better place. Read about these groundbreaking Canadian athletes who achieved their own dreams. They have also worked hard to help others do the same.

# Better Place

## Charmaine Crooks

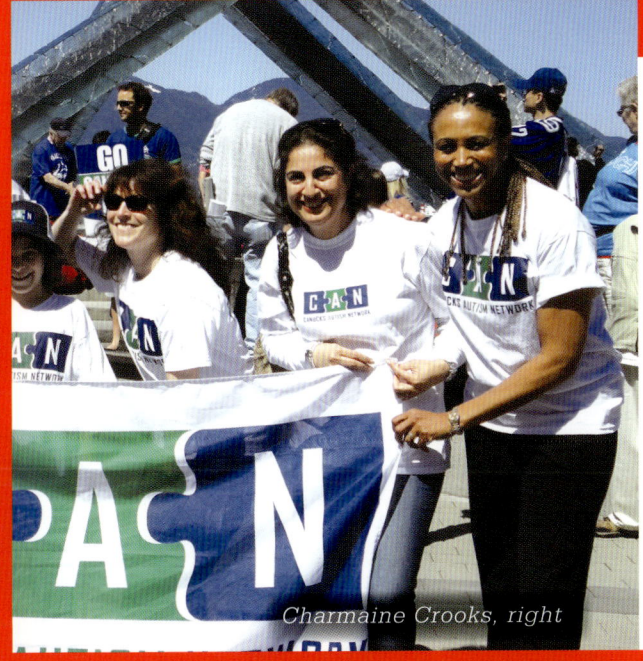
Charmaine Crooks, right

Charmaine Crooks was the first Canadian female athlete in track and field history to compete at five Olympic Games. She was also the first Canadian woman of colour to be a member of the International Olympic Committee. Crooks is equally successful off the track. After retiring from competitive sports, she founded a consulting group called NGU Consultants. Crooks is also passionate about volunteering. She volunteers for a number of local and global charities that focus on health, women, and youth. She is also involved with Right To Play. Through her volunteer work, she works to raise awareness about autism, heart disease, and breast cancer.

## Israel Idonije

Originally from Nigeria, Israel Idonije's family moved to Brandon, Manitoba, when he was four. Idonije played in the National Football League (NFL) for more than 10 years, and even made it to the Super Bowl. He also played for the Chicago Bears and the New York Giants. In 2007, Idonije started the Israel Idonije Foundation. The goal of the foundation is to help underprivileged children see their own potential and to help them set goals for their lives. The foundation runs camps for children in Winnipeg, Chicago, and West Africa (the three locations Idonije calls home).

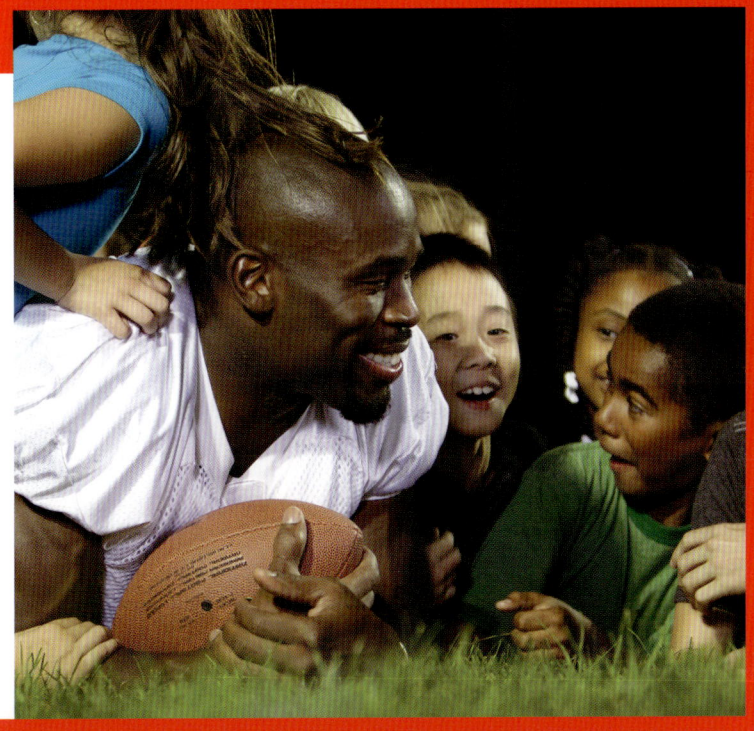

## Herb Carnegie

Herb Carnegie has been called the best Black hockey player never to play in the NHL. Although he was an amazing hockey player, he was offered a position on a farm team only. There was an unwritten rule at the time that said Black players couldn't play in the NHL. This didn't stop him from playing semi-professional hockey in the Quebec Provincial Hockey League with his brother, Ossie. They formed the first all-Black line, called the "Black Aces." After retiring, Carnegie went on to found the Herbert H. Carnegie Future Aces Foundation, as well as Canada's first hockey school. The foundation's mission is to empower young athletes both athletically and academically. Carnegie died in 2012.

farm team: *minor league team*
line: *group of players that all play together on the ice at the same time (left wing, centre, right wing)*

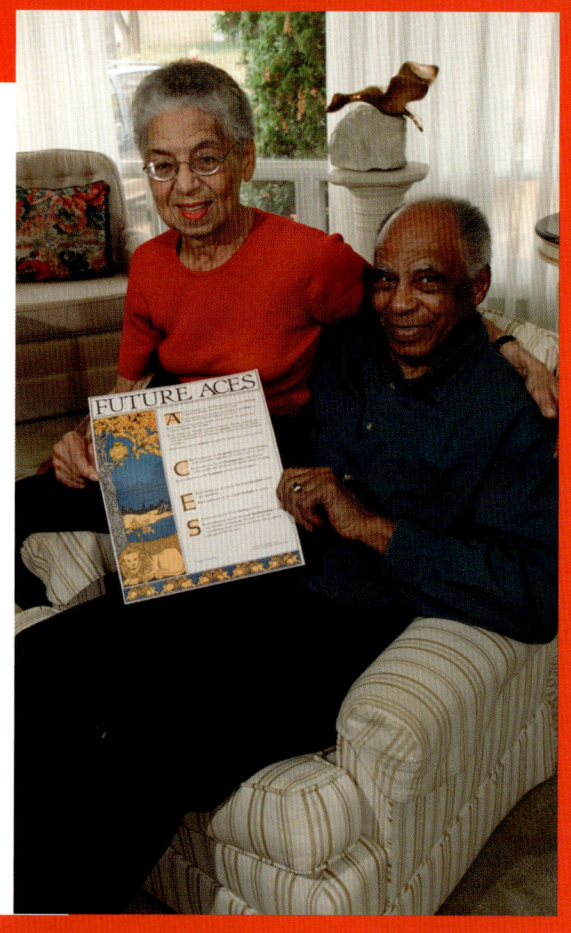

## Barb Howard

Barb Howard was the first African Canadian female to compete in an international competition. She won both a silver and a bronze medal for sprinting at the 1938 British Empire Games in Australia. Unfortunately, Howard's impressive athletic career was cut short due to the start of World War II. Because of the war, the 1940 Olympic Games were cancelled. Howard then decided to finish her education, eventually becoming a physical education teacher. In 1941, she became the first person of colour to be a teacher in Vancouver. She retired in 1984. During her time as a teacher, Howard worked at five elementary schools in Vancouver. She taught physical education to students with special needs.

## Fergie Jenkins

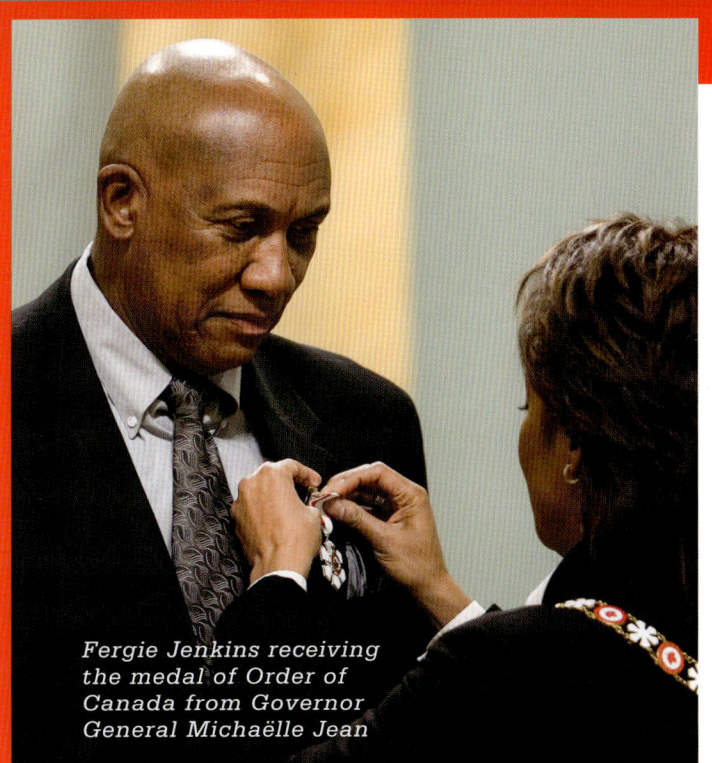

Fergie Jenkins receiving the medal of Order of Canada from Governor General Michaëlle Jean

In 1965, baseball player Fergie Jenkins was just 15. He was living in Chatham, Ontario. This is when he was scouted by the Philadelphia Phillies. In 1971, Jenkins won the National League's Cy Young Award. The award is given to the league's top pitcher. He is one of only four pitchers in Major League Baseball history to strike out 3000 batters while giving up fewer than 1000 walks. He is the only Canadian to ever be elected to the National Baseball Hall of Fame in Cooperstown, New York. The Fergie Jenkins Foundation was founded in 1997. Today, it raises money for over 500 charities in Canada and the United States. Jenkins was awarded the Order of Canada in 2007.

## Lennox Lewis

Boxer Lennox Lewis was born in London, England. His family moved to Canada when he was 12 years old. By the time he was 18, he was representing Canada at the Olympics. Although he didn't win a medal in his first Olympic Games, he took home a gold medal at the Olympic Games in Seoul in 1988. Lewis went on to become a professional boxer, and became the heavyweight champion in 1992. Lewis was inducted into the World Boxing Hall of Fame in 2008. He was inducted into the International Boxing Hall of Fame in 2009. Lewis created the Lennox Lewis League of Champions Foundation. The foundation's aim is to help disadvantaged kids in Canada, the United Kingdom, the United States, and Jamaica. The foundation works to help kids understand that success can be achieved through hard work, sacrifice, and believing in oneself.

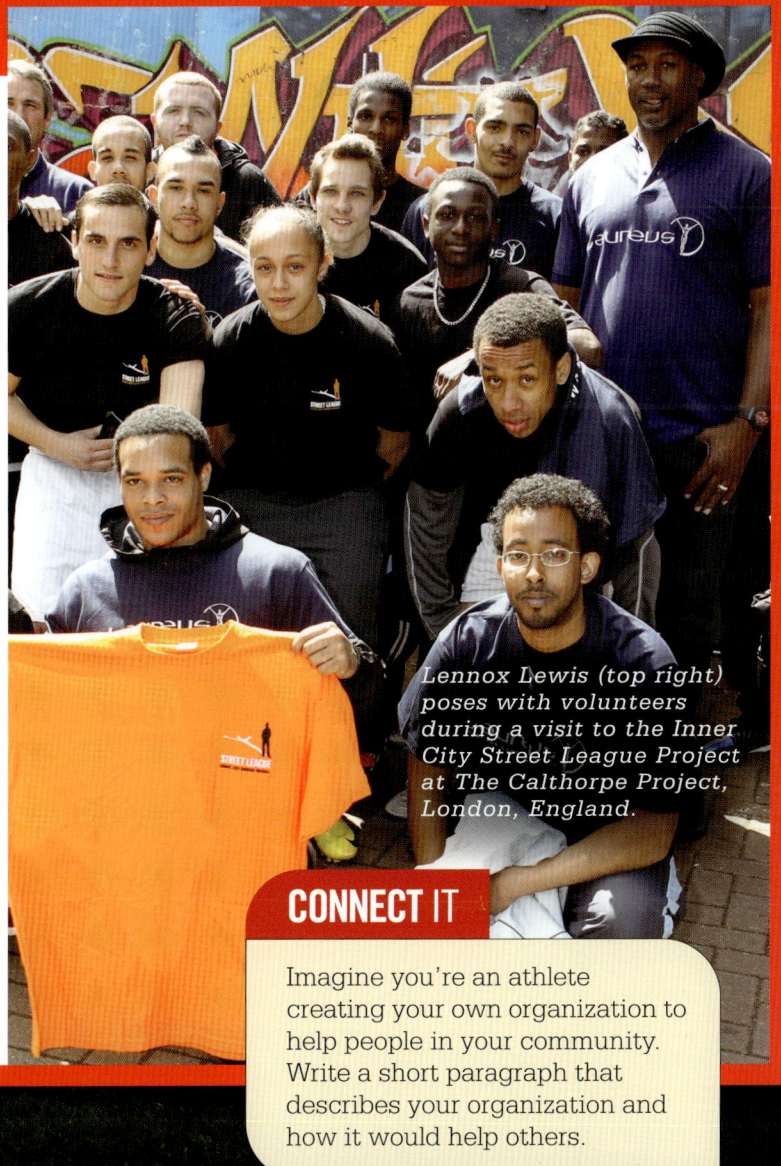

Lennox Lewis (top right) poses with volunteers during a visit to the Inner City Street League Project at The Calthorpe Project, London, England.

### CONNECT IT

Imagine you're an athlete creating your own organization to help people in your community. Write a short paragraph that describes your organization and how it would help others.

# The DREAM

### BY COREY GRANT

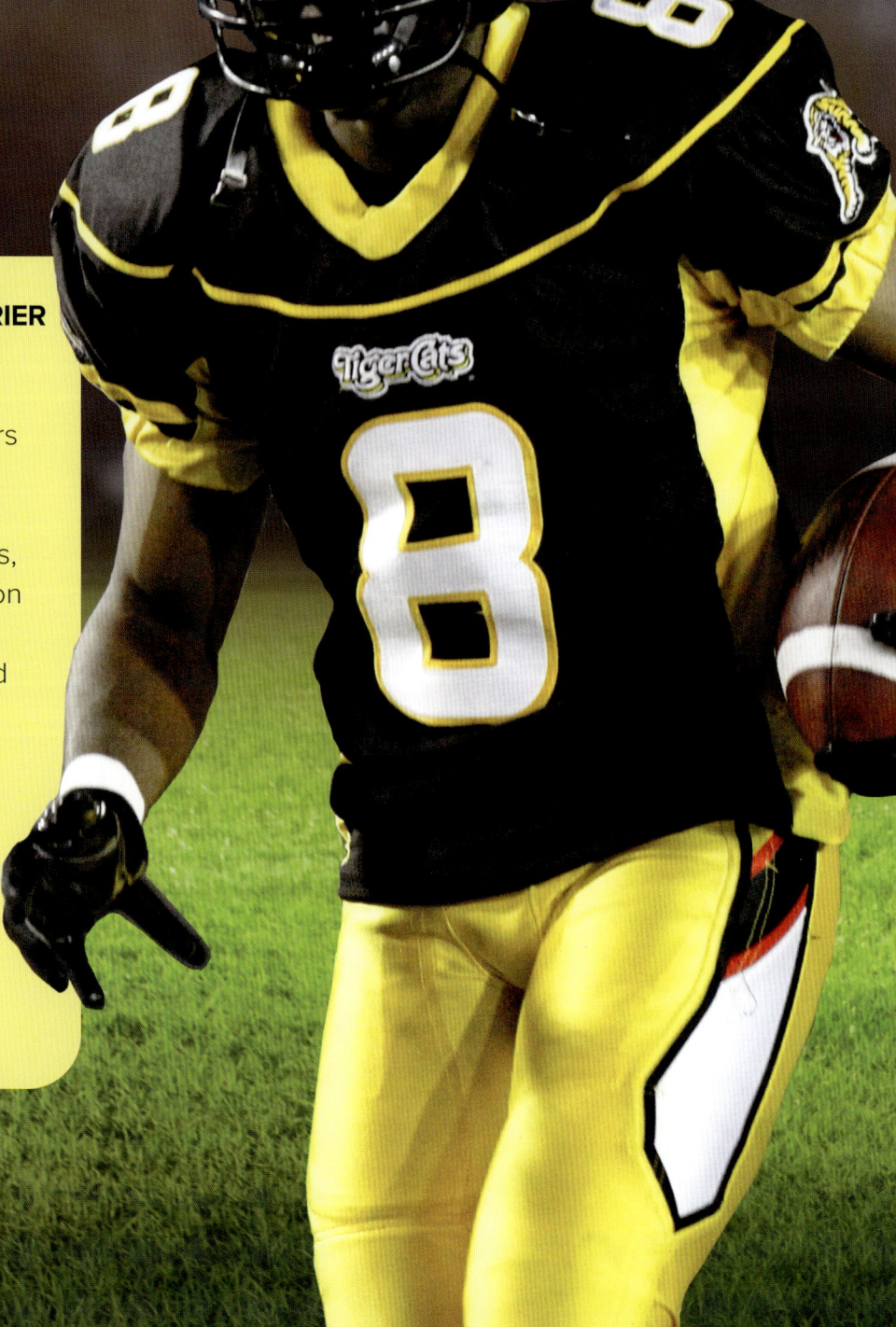

## THINK ABOUT IT

What advice would you give to someone who wants to pursue a career in sports?

**AFTER ATTENDING WILFRID LAURIER** University, Corey Grant was drafted seventh overall into the Canadian Football League (CFL). In the 11 years he played professional football, Grant played for the Saskatchewan Roughriders, the Montreal Alouettes, and the Hamilton Tiger-Cats. He won the Grey Cup with the Hamilton Tiger-Cats in his rookie season, and again with the Roughriders in 2007. He is now a coach for the Hamilton Tiger-Cats. He lives in Hamilton, Ontario, with his wife and two children. Before becoming a professional football coach in the CFL, he was an elementary school teacher with the Hamilton-Wentworth District School Board.

There was once a young author with a dream. This is what he wrote:

"My dream is to be a football player and play for the Hamilton Tiger-Cats. That may not happen, though, because I have only played football once. My dad told me if I got hurt, I wouldn't be able to play again, so instead of football, I would like to play hockey. But there is another small problem. I am not a good skater! So I guess I can't play hockey. If I do get a chance to play football, I want to be a quarterback because I have a good throw. I would get paid $240,000 a game, and I would be famous! When walking down the street, everyone would be cheering 'Corey! Corey' My nickname would be 'Awesome.' I would get tons of fan mail and answer every letter that I could. There would even be a statue of me! After I retired, I would be remembered for great plays. That's my dream."

I was that author. In grade 6, my teacher asked the class to create a "Book About Me." When I wrote my dream of becoming a professional football player and to play for the Hamilton Tiger-Cats, I knew I would have to make some difficult choices along the way. It wasn't going to be easy to achieve my dream.

As I chased my dream, I had to make many different sacrifices. Sometimes, I couldn't go out with friends because I had to train. I had to stay away from junk food because I knew it would affect my body and keep me from accomplishing my dream. As I got older, I started to realize how important it was to do well in school. The only way professional football teams would see me was by playing four years of university football. I wasn't the best student, so I had to work extra hard in ALL my classes. I made sure to ask for help when I needed help writing papers. I studied for tests and even stayed late for extra help. If I wanted to accomplish my dream of becoming a football player, I knew I had to do well in school, and I did.

I graduated from Wilfrid Laurier University. I was drafted in the first round by the Hamilton Tiger-Cats. Over the 11 years that I played in the CFL, I won two Grey Cups and was named Rookie of the Year for the Hamilton Tiger-Cats. I represented the Eastern Division as the CFL Rookie of the Year. I had accomplished my dream!

I accomplished my dream not solely because I wrote it down in grade 6. I believe I did it because I worked hard, stayed focused, and made sure I had great people around who supported me and kept me focused. If I can do it, anyone can do it, as long as you're willing to put in the work and make the necessary sacrifices to achieve your dream. I used these same methods to accomplish another dream of becoming a coach in the CFL. Now, I get to do a job that I love!

As Confucius said, "Do what you love, and you'll never have to work a day in your life."

## CONNECT IT

Research one of your role models. What was his or her dream? How did he or she overcome obstacles in order to achieve it? Write a journal entry in the voice of this person.

# Index

# Acknowledgements

Brand, Dionne. "Tuesday," from *Earth Magic*, written by Dionne Brand and illustrated by Eugenie Fernande. Used by permission of Kids Can Press Ltd. Toronto. Text © 1979, 2006 Dionne Brand.

Grant, Corey. "The Dream." Permission courtesy of the author.

Smith, Charles R. Jr. "Crack-Crack-Crunch," from *Winning Words: Sports Stories and Photographs*. Copyright © 2008 by Charles R. Smith Jr. Reproduced by permission of the publisher Candlewick Press, Somerville, MA.

Vogl, John. Excerpt from "Diversity Increasing, Minorities Shifting NHL Demographics," from *The Buffalo News*, 26 Jun. 2013. Permission courtesy of the author.

**Photo Sources**
**Cover:** whistle–BortN66/Shutterstock.com; **4:** [blue speed lines–wongwean; runner–Mark Herreid] Shutterstock.com; **6:** sports background–Jeremy Brooks; Lucy Diggs–Archives Center, National Museum of American History, Smithsonian Institution; Harlem Globetrotters–Harlem Globetrotters International, Inc; [Africville Sea-Sides; baseball team] Tom Connors/Nova Scotia Archives; **7:** Jackie Robinson–ClassicStock.com / Superstock; Althea Gibson–Palumbo, Fred/ Library of Congress; Willie O'Ree–AP Photo/CP Images; **8:** Abebe Bikila–Marka / SuperStock; Lusia Harris–Walter Iooss Jr. / Contributor / Getty Images; Ernie Davis–AP Photo/Jack Harris, File/ CP Images; Muhammad Ali–Glow Images / Keystone Archives; **9:** Jarome Iginla–Patrick Tuohy/ Shutterstock.com; Kevin Weekes–Jay Kopinski/Icon SMI 182/Jay Kopinski/Icon SMI/Newscom; Daniel Igali–Marco Chiesa UPI Photo Service/Newscom; Angela James–Images Distribution/ Agence Quebec Presse/Newscom; P.K. Subban–Fanny Schertzer; **10:** [ribbons–TatjanaRittner; medal–AlexRoz] Shutterstock.com; **11:** torchbearers–ZUMAPRESS.com/Keystone Press; **12:** track field–gopause/Shutterstock.com; Ian Sheppard–courtesy of Ian Sheppard; **13:** Peter Snider– John Sims, Team Ontario/Nancy Snider; Monique Shah–Special Olympics Ontario/June Shah; **14:** [background–vs148; puck–mexrix] Shutterstock.com; Seth Jones, Darnell Nurse–Graig Abel / Contributor / Getty Images; ice–SebStock/Shutterstock.com; **15:** Darnell Nurse–Anne-Marie Sorvin/USA TODAY Sports; Seth Jones–Sergei Belski/USA TODAY Sports; **16:** Willie O'Ree–Gregg Forwerck / Stringer / Getty Images; **17:** Jonathan-Ismael Diaby–Richard Wolowicz / Contributor / Getty Images; **18:** [houses–imagesef; sky–Serg64] Shutterstock.com; Dionne Brand–Fred Lum / The Globe and Mail/CP Images; girl–Megan Little; **20:** illustrations–Megan Little; background– Evgeny Karandaev/Shutterstock.com; **23:** [web–Gandras; tech border–URRRA; phone–photka] Shutterstock.com; **24:** [sand texture–Piotr Grzymkowski; watercolor–donatas1205] Shutterstock. com; **25:** [chess piece–Ognian; car–dmitriylo; pool balls–Jason Winter; pool cue–Jiripravda; Mancala–matabum] Shutterstock.com; senet–Keith Schengili-Roberts; **26:** [marbles–STILLFX; animals–Vector pro; man–CREATISTA; girl–Diego Cervo] Shutterstock.com; **27:** Morabaraba board–adamoell; controller–Nata-Lia/Shutterstock.com; **28:** Ferguson Jenkins Jr.–Malcolm Emmons/USA TODAY Sports; Michael Jordan–RVR Photos/USA TODAY Sports; **29:** Serena Williams–lev radin/Shutterstock.com; Jesse Owens–iStockphoto.com/© Ken Brown; Willie O'Ree–B Bennett / Contributor / Getty Images; **30:** Charmaine Crooks–CP PHOTO/ COC/ Claus Andersen; Bruny Surin–Claus Andersen UPI Photo Service/Newscom; Muhammad Ali–topham Picturepoint / GetStock.com; **31:** background–javarman/Shutterstock.com; Perdita Felicien–Tony Bock / Toronto Star / GetStock.com; **32:** Perdita Felicien–JEFF HAYNES / Staff / Getty Images; **33:** Perdita Felicien–THE CANADIAN PRESS/Aaron Vincent Elkaim; **34:** illustrations–Leisl Adams; **39:** [background–Lurin; pommel horse–Alexander Ishchenko] Shutterstock.com; Curtis Hibbert 1988– PC Photo/AOC/CP Images; Curtis Hibbert 1992–PC Photo/AOC/CP Images; **40:** sports field–winui/ Shutterstock.com; Nelson Mandela–KIM LUDBROOK/EPA/Newscom; **41:** Mandela, Pienaar–imago sportfotodienst/Newscom; **42:** [sports field–wavebreakmedia; trophy–doomu] Shutterstock.com; **43:** Charmaine Crooks–Canucks Autism Network/Lindsau Petrie; Israel Idonije & Kids–Play 60 Cadence Health via the Israel Idonije Foundation; **44:** Herb Carnegie and wife–David Cooper / GetStock.com; Barb Howard–Rebecca Bollwitt; **45:** Fergie Jenkins–CP PHOTO/Fred Charrand; Lennox Lewis and kids–PLAA/ZDS WENN Photos/Newscom; **46:** stadium–winui/Shutterstock. com; Corey Grant–courtesy of Corey Grant.